D0872279

TARGET:
CANCER

Also by the author

THE GENE AGE:
GENETIC ENGINEERING
AND THE NEXT INDUSTRIAL REVOLUTION
(WITH CO-AUTHOR LYNN C. KLOTZ)

TARGET: CANCER

Edward J. Sylvester

CHARLES SCRIBNER'S SONS

New York

For Ginny, with love

Copyright © 1986 Edward J. Sylvester

Library of Congress Cataloging-in-Publication Data

Sylvester, Edward J.
Target—cancer.

Includes index.
1. Cancer—Popular works. 2. Cancer—Research—
Popular works. I. Title. [DNLM: 1. Neoplasms.
QZ 200 S97695t]
RC263.S987   1986   616.99′4   85-22089
ISBN 0-684-18478-8

Published simultaneously in Canada by Collier Macmillan Canada, Inc.
Copyright under the Berne Convention.

All rights reserved.
No part of this book may be reproduced
in any form without the permission
of Charles Scribner's Sons.

1 3 5 7 9 11 13 15 17 19   F/C   20 18 16 14 12 10 8 6 4 2

Printed in the United States of America.

Contents

Acknowledgements

A book like this is necessarily the product of many people's efforts. Many of those who have made significant contributions are quoted in the text and, even though their roles were often far more important than they may appear, they are at least acknowledged there. Others played a major part in my education in the intricacies of the world reported here, yet they do not appear in the text.

At the National Cancer Institute, I am most indebted to the tireless efforts of Joyce Doherty, the complete-professional information officer who helped arrange interviews and provided guidance on where to turn for information; and to Conrad Storad, former Arizona State University graduate assistant, NCI fellow, and now a Kent State University information staffer, a fine science writer himself whose efforts in giving me background were invaluable.

Many medical scientists at the NCI granted often-extensive interviews that contributed significantly to my knowledge, and I am very grateful for their time: Curt Harris, Thomas Waldmann, Alan Rabson, George VandeWoude, Mariano Barbacid, Jeff Schlom, Ira Pastan, Elizabeth Weisberger, Sam Broder, Stuart Aaronson, Peter Greenwald, Robert Ozols, Charles Myers, Bruce Chabner, Eli Gladstein and Gilbert Jay.

At the University of Arizona, information officer Ruth Iliff was most helpful in arranging interviews and in getting me background information. I am also indebted to the scientists and medical personnel of the Cancer Center, especially Laurie Young, Rail Robertson, Robert Heusinkveld, and Jeff Trent.

At MD Anderson, members of the information staff were very

helpful, and I appreciate the interviews with such medical scientists as Lee Murray, Peter Almond, Kenneth McCredie and Douglas Vizard.

In Boston and Cambridge, where most of this book takes place, the aid I received was both extensive and varied. I owe a great debt of gratitude to Lois Kessin, whose generosity with her time and energy left me more of both to devote to this book, and to Robert Bensetler for his generosity in housing the wandering writer. To Mitch and Jane Goroski, I am grateful for an illuminating conversation that helped direct this book.

At Dana-Farber Cancer Institute, many thanks to the information office, and especially to Karen Gregory of the breast-cancer clinic for guidance and assistance in setting up interviews.

Special thanks to Barbara Cahill, Robert Weinberg's secretary, for her frequent, generous assistance.

I am especially indebted to BioTechnica International, the Cambridge genetic engineering firm, for the use of office space, telephone and, most important to me, the camaraderie of its terrific staff during a long summer's work.

Back home at Arizona State University, producing this book was immeasurably easier thanks to the efforts of Sandra Colombo, executive director of the University Program for Faculty Development, and Kathleen Milbrandt, her assistant. Their Microcomputer Resource Facility became my writing haven; more important, they and their assistants were my source of endless advice and information on what, just a year ago, seemed impenetrable and now is familiar: word-processing with WordStar, with which this book was written and indexed.

Finally, I thank the ASU College of Public Programs and Dean Nicholas Henry, and the Walter Cronkite School of Journalism and Telecommunication and Director ElDean Bennett for the time to carry out this project.

***

The fine illustrations are the work of May S. Cheney of BioCommunications, Phoenix, Arizona.

***

This book would not have been possible without the financial assistance of Mrs. Lila Morris, to whom I am deeply grateful.

Prologue

What is cancer? We have had this killer with us as far back in time as we can see. Its markings dot and score Stone Age bones; it was treated surgically in ancient Egypt; was called *carcinos* by Hippocrates the Greek, cancer by the Romans, both names referring to one of the deadliest traits of the disease: the crablike appearance of a tumor that has begun reaching out arms to invade other tissue of the body.

Cancer will be responsible for one in four American deaths this year unless, by the time you read this, something near miraculous has happened. Cancer is treatable—certainly more so than twenty years ago. Treatment extends life, often cures the rare cancers, and occasionally cures the most prevalent; but the overall death rate from cancer has changed remarkably little in our time.

But what *is* it? Until very recently that question was as frustratingly unanswerable as efforts to cure the disease were frustratingly unsuccessful. This story is about some remarkable discoveries made over the past decade that have begun to answer that ages-old question—finally, definitively. The impetus of this book was an accumulation of reports from friends in science that researchers were beginning to solve one part of cancer's riddle. They are learning, step by step, what happens in the conversion of ordinary human cells to cancerous cells. My aim was to find out what was known of this most feared disease, because lacking that, how do you tell a coherent story of the hunt for its cure? How do you look for something if you don't know what it is you're looking for? That paradox, put forth by Plato nearly 2,500 years ago, would raise its head again and again as I tried to learn where we stand on the road to conquering cancer. *What is cancer?* many doctors would ask. *Tell me what it is and I'll tell you where we stand.* And it is a challenge that doctors regularly put to scientists who claim to have unraveled yet another secret of cancer. This, I quickly found out, was no mean challenge, the answers emerging no easy answers.

I set out to interview doctors, patients, and scientists because the likeliest place to go for answers was to those most intimately involved in cancer, and in the most radically different ways.

The story of the encircling of this ancient scourge marks the very latest developments in molecular biology, which, with its attendant specialties, seems to be emerging as the dominant science of the latter half of the twentieth century—certainly in the public imagination, with the development of genetic engineering and newly revealed "secrets of life," but equally in its position at center stage in the world's leading scientific journals.

The British journal *Nature*, which covers as broad a spectrum of the sciences as its name implies, is now largely devoted to molecular biology and related life sciences, in both text and advertising. Its editor, John Maddox, a physicist, confessed to me that he would be happy to see discoveries in physics find an equal place in the journal but generally was quite happy that it was cornering the best of recent biological discoveries. We were speaking during a break in a Boston conference sponsored by *Nature*: "The Molecular Biology of Cancer." During the closing moments of that conference Maddox hailed the U.S. government's support for research into the causes and cures of cancer as "magnificent . . . second to none in the world."

And that, of course, would play a key role in this story—the quantity and quality of the federal effort to conquer cancer. Although federal involvement in cancer research goes back half a century, the large-scale "war against cancer" truly began with passage of the 1971 National Cancer Act, which, among other things, designated the National Cancer Institute (NCI) a separate arm of the National Institutes of Health. Since then the NCI has always been well funded, but recent cutbacks have thrown some of the best researchers' efforts into near disarray, another element of the story that would emerge.

Cancer is more than a disease; it is a powerful social force. Its effects are very different from those of the terrible epidemic diseases of the past, for it is not an epidemic; but as this story unfolds it will become clear that its effects are no less universal. Billions are spent on research, even more billions on treatment for what a respected surgeon in Tucson would confess is often "a very, very expensive form of psychotherapy," when costly treatments are applied to those who cannot be helped—but cannot be abandoned. More troublesome, a noted cancer specialist in Boston said he believed that if some simple and inexpensive replacement for chemotherapy for the treatment of cancer were found tomorrow, all U.S. medical schools would teeter on the verge of bankruptcy, so integral a part of their hospital revenues is oncology, the medical specialty of cancer treatment.

Strange, then, that a disease so widespread in its effects, so feared, should be so little understood. At one time it will seem a single thing to be given that single name, at another a group of diseases with little commonality and the more frightening for that reason. There are sarcomas and carcinomas, the broadest distinction of type; the latter account for nearly 90 percent of all cancers, those of the epithelial tissue that forms the skin and the linings of all major organs. Sarcomas attack the connective tissue: bone, cartilage, striated (voluntary) muscle. There are also brain tumors, liver cancers, two entirely different kinds of breast cancer, lung and stomach cancers, and leukemias, the cancers of the blood. There is teratocarcinoma, "the monster," named because its tumor appears like an animal growing within, and Hodgkin's disease, a lymphoma (cancer of the lymph system) that attacks young people and old people and almost no one in between. Some two hundred forms of cancer have been distinguished. It has more names than the devil and seems as good at changing place and appearance.

All cancers have two things in common: uncontrolled growth—cells growing and dividing without end, which animal cells are not supposed to do—and the ability of cancer cells to migrate to neighboring and finally distant sites, a step that marks first invasion and then the deadly stage called metastasis. Different kinds of cancer do not behave alike; worse, in two patients the same kind of tumor will behave in radically different ways. One patient may be cured, another may die, still another may appear disease free for years only to have a recurrence.

Thus, getting a grip on what cancer is seems as complicated as understanding life and death. Just as it seems pinpointed it will suddenly appear a vague, generalized comment on the human body's behavior, the common cold tuned up to a deadly intensity, a consequence of stress like an ulcer or high blood pressure, an effect of negative thought to be cured by right thinking. The word changes color and texture before your eyes, like a landscape in different lights, and so seems to change its nature.

But just as many top scientists were ready to accept that answer that there was no answer, a decade ago an answer began to emerge, and that is what this book is about: an emerging answer tantalizingly half complete, a figure half light and half darkness. Even though we have not identified the killer, we know we are close. Not to a single thing, perhaps, but to a common form, a pattern; we have found what one scientist called a funnel, a vortex. All the diverse and seemingly unrelated facts about cancer appear to come down to a few basic principles, and that means there *will* one day be an answer.

The killer certainly has not been caught. The most deadly cancers in the United States—lung cancer, postmenopausal breast cancer, and colorectal cancers—are no more curable now than thirty to forty years ago, when surgery, radiation, and chemotherapy were first making their marks as combined regimens, although people with these cancers in some cases are surviving longer. That is my conclusion after speaking to many people who are expert in a subject of much dispute: the success of the war against cancer. Dramatic forms of cancer now can be cured—the most common childhood cancers and testicular cancer, for example—but they are rare compared to the major three killers in America, or to such scourges in other parts of the world as liver and stomach cancer.

Down through the ages this forbidding star of an outreaching tumor mass has been seen through the glass of the most sophisticated medical science of its time—and that science often was later found flawed. To look for something you must first have an idea of what *it* is. Now watch this evolution of an idea.

The Greek physician saw a crablike tumor mass and surgically removed it, a fixed, finite, if growing thing. Much later, the Roman physician Galen believed cancer to be caused by "humours" that circulated through the body; through the lens of this theory he correctly accounted for the systemic nature of the disease—that it spreads through the system and is not confined to the original tumor's location. And through this lens he failed to see that cancer often could be corrected surgically. It was not until the eighteenth century that the Greek and early Roman practice of cancer surgery resumed.

In the early nineteenth century, when the French physician Recamier suggested that new tumors were "metastases," distant colonies of the original tumor, he was ridiculed, although this turned out to be absolutely correct. But at that time the medical community was just confronting the infectious nature of so much disease, and the proponents of the idea that microbes were responsible for infection had just won out over those who had previously ridiculed them. Cancer was believed to be yet another disease for which an infectious agent would soon be found.

That idea fell into disrepute only to enjoy a major renaissance in the middle of this century with the rise of the science of virology, the study of viruses. Many viruses were found to cause cancers in animals (after the biologist who made this discovery was ignored for many years), and it seemed virtually certain that the viral origin of human cancers would ultimately be proven.

Each of these notions has proved to have elements of truth and has revealed or accounted for some facet of the disease, and that is why our ideas about cancer today are truly evolutionary. Yet none of the historical notions accounted for the enormous complexity of the disease, and that is why the discoveries that form the immediate background to this story are of such importance. They pointed toward a simple, discrete number of events that would account for *oncogenesis*, the onset of cancer.

Considering how the views of cancer have reflected historical periods, how characteristic it is of the twentieth-century American way of doing things in a big way that we have "declared war" on cancer, and to that end have thrown massive technological, human, and financial resources, and awe-inspiring energy, into defeating "the enemy." And in one respect this declaration was quite apt. The development of warfare over the millennia has, however unfortunately, mirrored the development and sophistication of human society. The war against cancer has grown and developed in scope and sophistication in just that way, mirroring the best we have had to offer in material resources and brainpower.

The United States is dotted with dozens of research–treatment centers, ranging from multibillion-dollar operations like those of the University of Texas System Cancer Center in Houston, the Dana-Farber Cancer Institute in Boston, and the National Cancer Institute in suburban Washington, to smaller but well-respected institutions like the Arizona Medical Center in Tucson. Those are the places that figure in my story. I could as easily have picked a number of others, heard the same hope and pain in the voices of patients and doctors, the same intensity and excitement in the voices of scientists.

This story is of an odyssey in the year 1984, a year that for more than forty years symbolized Orwellian doom in a world stifled and controlled by perfected totalitarianism, a year that for me was a time of discovery in a decade of immeasurably important discoveries concerning the causes and cures of cancer. And I like the irony of that year's connotation.

George Orwell's novel 1984, a personal favorite, has always seemed to me more classical tragedy than it is credited for being. Such tragedies need giant, heroic figures, destroyed by fate. And the heroic figure of 1984 is: thinking. Not flat and abstract "thought," but the powerful, disputatious, determined, ever-hungry thinking we so admire in Western culture. To the Greeks, the active verb "to think" had at its root logos, seen by the ancients as the all-powerful driving force of the universe, not the truly lazy and comfortable activity we sometimes let ourselves see it as. In 1984, that kind of thinking is dead. In 1984 it was alive and kicking: in Tucson, where a young girl talked of her certainty that she would live free of Hodgkins' disease; in Houston, where a world-famous oncologist argued forcefully against letting cancer, the killer, be abstracted into a laboratory notion; at the NCI, where an unorthodox and criticized scientist had found a human cancer virus after most others had given up the search; in Cambridge, Massachusetts, and Cold Spring Harbor, New York, where a handful of scientists, obscure outside their own disciplines, changed a century's way of looking at cancer within the space of a few years.

Odyssey. For me a voyage of discovery, but some distinction is needed. Odysseus was just trying to get home when he became the hero of his epic. I left home, near Phoenix, looking for something, for some answers. I am the only person in this story who is *not* a protagonist; those who provided the answers are—and they are as wide-ranging and talented a group of people as one would expect in a multidimensional world like that of cancer. It is a world resolvable into three primary dimensions.

The victims. They are children in a Boston clinic, survivors of ordeals more painful than their parents have endured, and they are their parents, who agonize. They are young adults just setting out, suddenly encountering the real and present threat of death. They are older people, cancer's most frequent victims. To them all, cancer is a thing completely personal, intimate, unwanted. At best it is a major force reshaping their lives and those of their families—though not always, interestingly, for the worse. *Cancer teaches the value and meaning of time,* the victim said. *I wouldn't go through it again; I'm not sorry I went through it.*

The doctors. However complex their efforts may be in dealing with cancer, what it *is* is brutally simple. *We see cancer as it comes through the door,* says the chief of medical oncology at one of the nation's major centers, defining a relationship at once intensely personal, full of highs and lows a doctor must learn to live with, yet detached. *It's hardest of all on the young residents, of course. They come in believing they can save people, then they have to watch people die. When they become too involved, they become less-good doctors. The patients don't want your sympathy, I tell them. They want you to be a doctor.*

The scientists. To some of the best minds in half a dozen different branches of biology, generally centered on molecular biology, cancer represents a personal quest that absorbs their waking thoughts, consumes their energies, defines their careers. The cancer search has become a scientific challenge exceeded by no other, one to match the quests for space flight, artificial intelligence, and the secrets of the atom. *What we're finding out when we study cancer is really about how life works,* the scientist said. Indeed, the fascination of the scientist with cancer is at base an obsession with learning the secrets of life—not of death, not even of disease per se.

The scientific dimension represents the dominant perspective in this story, not arbitrarily. The cure for the major life-threatening cancers may or may not be close. Human suffering, courage, and failure, like Heraclitus' river, do not change yet are new with their every expression. But major discoveries have brought excitement and optimism to cancer research, the very dimension of the cancer world that just a few years ago offered the most pessimistic view. And along this axis, at last, we can begin to see what it is we are talking about.

It is in this dimension that several other people enter as much as collaborators as sources, although they will be seen in the course of the story in their roles as scientists. Lynn Klotz, vice president for developing new businesses for the Cambridge genetic engineering firm Bio-Technica International, is a former associate professor in Harvard's department of biochemistry and molecular biology. While there he was a teacher of Paula Traktman; and he was a colleague of Lew Cantley, whose perceptions of the state of cancer research proved vital and whose own work, unexpectedly for me, would prove of singular importance within the story. Klotz was advisor to graduate student Tom Roberts, whose chance encounter with Cantley on the street would begin an important scientific collaboration seen in the end of the story; he was also a teacher of Michael Kriegler: *I don't want to take baby steps,* Kriegler would say. *If I fail, fine, but I'm going to try to do something important.*

Traktman, her perceptions always acute, explained much of the background so important to understanding where science is now in cancer research. A graduate student with Nobel laureate David Baltimore, she became a good friend of Robert Weinberg, Huki Land, Luis Parada, Cliff Tabin, and Mitch Goldfarb, names that emerge from many other sources in key roles in the developing idea of "oncogenes," genes that cause cancer by their inappropriate actions within the human cell.

Cantley and wife Vicki Sato guided and steered me on this journey, where tiny deviations of language, like small misreadings of the compass, can lead straight to rocks and whirlpools. Cantley, seen here as an associate professor at Harvard, is now a full professor at Tufts Medical School. Sato, his and Klotz's former colleague at Harvard, is director of cell biology and immunology for Biogen, one of the world's largest genetic engineering firms and a leading manufacturer of interferon, a substance being tested in clinical trials around the country for antitumor activity. She is an immunologist, her specialty perhaps the least understood in its relationship to cancer, although one that virtually all scientists believe must play a key role if cancer is to be prevented or cured.

The odyssey. *What causes cancer? What is cancer?* Head south from Phoenix on a scorching May day, to Arizona Medical Center in Tucson. *What can you do? You cannot tell someone, I can do nothing more for you. People cannot stand to hear that; they must have some hope.* Turn east to Houston, to M.D. Anderson Hospital and its sprawling research and treatment facilities. *All progress is made in the clinic. In the clinic, where the patients are, in the clinic where you see cancer.* And north to Bethesda, Maryland, just shy of Washington. *We hope to cut the cancer-death rate in half by the year 2000.* That's the goal set by Vincent DeVita, director of the National Cancer Institute. Northward still to Boston and Cambridge.

There, except for short trips, I stayed through mid-September, when *Nature* providentially hosted its conference on cancer, bringing together many of the best-known cancer researchers and physicians, many of whom by then were familiar faces. Boston–Cambridge: *There's no place like this. This is probably the most exciting research environment in the world. Harvard, MIT, all the hospitals like Dana-Farber, Children's, on and on.*

On and on. Of course, the story doesn't end there.

PART I

DARK STARS

1

The Bridge

Mid-February, 1978, a bitter late afternoon already dark. Robert Weinberg is making his way across Longfellow Bridge, walking the few miles from his laboratory in the Massachusetts Institute of Technology's cancer institute to his home in Boston's Beacon Hill section because snow has paralyzed all transportation. He has often skied to and from school, even on good days, but today is stuck on foot, and the plows have peeled back the snow blanket into furls across the sidewalk so he has to clamber and posthole his way across the Charles River, frozen solid below the bridge.

This is no time for a great notion, but it comes. The idea lights up his mind as though all the notions and worries banging around in his head had finally reached a critical point of chain reaction, so the idea bursts and coalesces. Sometimes people pursue great ideas with no single moment identifiable when "it" occurred to them "that . . ." And sometimes, as now, the moment when a person's life takes off is singular and memorable in fine detail. He has just thought of the experiment, and as quickly as it comes to him he is utterly convinced it will work.

A major controversy raged in molecular biology through the 1970s, one that has not completely ended, and although the causes of cancer were at the root of it the battle lines were drawn much more broadly, dividing scientists of various disciplines within molecular biology—

3

the science that studies living systems at the molecular level of their operation. Three key concepts were involved, still the key concepts in the field of cancer research: genes and genetics, viruses, and chemical carcinogens. All virtually buzzwords to even the casual newspaper reader, in science these names label whole continents of complex theories, years' worth of experiments and mountains of scientific data.

For the moment, let's target only the broadest definitions of these: As has been known for a half century, the units of inheritance of all living things on earth are located on a long chemical molecule called deoxyribonucleic acid, or DNA (see Figure 1). Those units were called genes long before biologists even knew what chemicals might be involved in inheritance, but now it is known that a gene corresponds to a piece of that DNA molecule.

Genetics, the study of inheritance that traditionally focused on the laws by which visible traits would be passed along from plant or animal organisms to their offspring, now has come down to the submicroscopic level. Here molecular genetics studies the chemical molecules involved in inheritance, growth, and reproduction. Classical genetics teaches us that as a growing cell reaches the point of dividing into two identical "daughter" cells, its chromosomes, tangled skeins of DNA, reproduce; half go to each daughter cell. By contrast, molecular genetics focuses on how the DNA molecule itself reproduces, or replicates, during this phase, with half the doubled DNA going to each daughter cell.

And viruses, of course, are those extraordinarily tiny compositions of the nucleic acid DNA or the related RNA (ribonucleic acid) wrapped in a bit of protein, which cause everything from the common cold to warts, and which have been implicated in cancer since early in this century. In fact, only toxic chemicals have been as frequently cited as the cause of cancer, chemicals ranging from the known carcinogens like asbestos and cigarette smoke to the suspect, like saccharine.

By early 1978, simply put, there were those who believed as Weinberg did that cancer was a disease rooted in the genetic part of the cell—the cell's nucleus, or command center, which contains the DNA, the genes. This group included many of America's leading scientists, and they had amassed a good amount of evidence to back their claim.

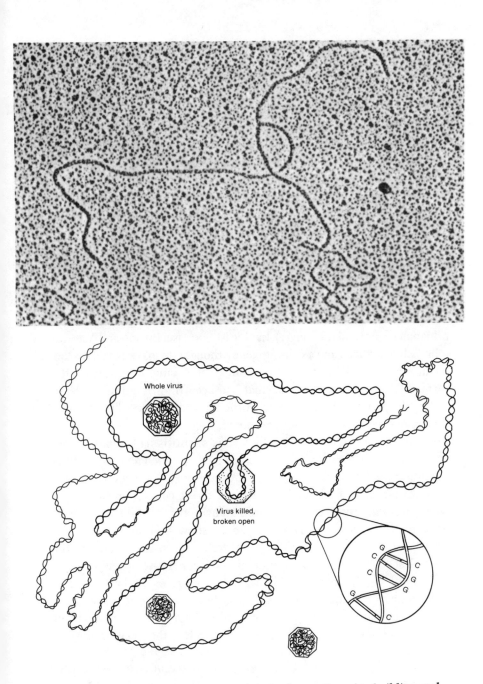

Figure 1. The DNA molecule contains the instructions for building and maintaining the living thing in which it is found. Top: Actual photo of a bacterial DNA molecule that has been "iced" with protein to make it visible under the electron microscope. Bottom: A lifelike rendering of animal viruses as they appear under the electron microscope. One virus has been chemically broken up so its DNA spews into the surrounding medium. If it could be further magnified, the DNA would be seen as a spiral staircase whose steps are a combination of four bases.

And there were those who offered powerful arguments to the contrary, and *they* included some of the best scientists in America.

Of the critics, some believed that cancer-causing genes might exist but were not an important part of the human cancer process; for example, such oncogenes might be a symptom rather than a cause of cancer, an aberration in gene structure that was a consequence of the disease and not the spark that fired it. The prefix *onco-* denotes cancer; thus oncogenes, although they had not been found, were by definition aberrant genes suspected of causing cancer, either by inheritance or by damage after birth.

Oncogenes had first been accurately described in 1975 by Michael Bishop and Harold Varmus, both M.D. researchers at the University of California at San Francisco and two of the country's leaders in virology. (The term virologist can apply to a wide range of researchers interested in viruses; the virologists in this story are all in a major branch of molecular biology.) In at least one case, Bishop and Varmus had shown that cancer-causing genes thought to have somehow become implanted in an infected animal by a virus were in fact the animal's own genes, but genes that had been thrown out of whack so they did not function properly. Although that is generally accepted now, in 1978 it was still hotly disputed.

After Bishop and Varmus's discovery, scientists had found further indications that cancer's basis was genetic, *independent* of whether viruses were involved. In the mid-1970s, Bruce Ames of the University of California at Berkeley had shown a direct correlation between a chemical's ability to cause cancer in animals and its ability to damage the genes of bacteria. That seemed to show that inducing cancer involved damaging genes. The Ames test, in fact, is still used as the simplest first indicator of whether a chemical is carcinogenic: If the chemical causes mutation, damage, to the genes of bacteria in a laboratory dish, that is taken as prima facie evidence it would cause cancer by damaging the genes of humans. But the major import of Ames's findings for scientists was to tighten the relationship between cancer and gene damage.

Virologists of this time were frequently at odds with those who argued that chemicals, not viruses, were the major cause of human cancers; it was seen as an "either/or" proposition. Viruses were long known to cause cancer in animals, and since the mid-1970s, virologists had been able routinely to infect animal cells in culture with cancer, via viruses, and those cells could be mixed with fresh batches of cells, which would similarly become infected by the viral cancer. *Transfection* would turn out to be singularly important in cancer research. In general, the word transfection simply refers to infecting an organism or cell with a suspected disease agent, then using some fragment of that organism or cell to infect others. In this case, animal cells infected with cancer viruses would induce cancer in uninfected colonies.

The problem: No virus had ever been found that would infect a human cell culture with cancer. Conversely, no human cancer patient had ever been found infected with a virus that could be associated with the disease.

In the broad sense of the word, "causes" of cancer have been known for years. In 1775, British physician Percival Pott reported that the testicular cancer commonplace among London chimney sweeps was caused by a chemical in coal soot. In fact, even before Pott a Scottish physician linked the use of snuff with cancers of the nose, mouth, and throat, two hundred years before the U.S. Surgeon General warned of the hazards of smoking. Early in this century it was found that x-rays could cause cancer, and everything from the ultraviolet rays of sunlight to chemicals in aniline dyes are known carcinogens—causes of cancer.

But that wasn't what Weinberg or other scientists meant by what "causes" cancer. They wanted to find the series of steps involved in oncogenesis—*onco* + *genesis,* cancer's creation or onset. Even many of those who believed that cancer had a genetic basis—that is, that it involved damage to the organism's genes, as the Ames test indicated—argued against the possibility that causes in this strict sense would ever be laid out. These critics contended that virtually any sharp "blow," chemical or otherwise, to almost any gene or genes might lead to cancer, that it might be a plague with causes virtually beyond limit. That idea makes a lot of common sense. The growth and development of all living things is determined by extremely precise controls and regulations embodied within the genes; it seemed quite plausible that any jolt to this precise machinery could send it spinning out of control, and uncontrolled growth is the hallmark of cancer cells.

But Weinberg did not believe that, nor was he alone. He believed that the number of steps in the transformation of a cell from normal to cancerous was limited and precise, and more importantly, that there was a common pattern in oncogenesis regardless of type of cancer or the affected organism.

This was an optimistic view: If the causes of cancers were limited, so might be the steps to prevent or cure the disease. Although there might be years between the finding of causes and the finding of cures, the description of these steps would certainly offer light at the end of the tunnel. But how to prove what Weinberg and others felt utterly convinced was true?

In general, on one side of this dispute were the virologists, like Weinberg and Bishop, who studied viruses not merely as disease-causing "agents," but in a more basic way, as models of how genes behave. Viruses are really just a small number of genes packaged in a protein coat. Because they are so extraordinarily simple, viruses offer a unique system for getting at the truths of elemental gene behavior. As Weinberg put it, viruses enabled scientists to watch genes operating outside the jungle of complexity that is the normal working environment for genes of higher animals.

On the other side were many cytologists—specialists in the internal organization of cells—and a good many medical researchers of various specialties, who saw much of the virologist's work as academic and obscure. They believed, to oversimplify the dispute, that the place to study mammalian genes was in mammalian cells; and that until the difficulties of doing so were overcome, there was little purpose in speaking of cancer-gene research.

The adversaries were fighting it out with the zeal, and sometimes the anger and bitterness, with which scientists often wage wars of ideas outside the public's ken and most often outside its interest. But this particular battle has a sharp twist. Viruses have been known to cause cancer in animals since 1911, when biologist Peyton Rous announced discovery of a virus that caused tumors in chickens. After years of skepticism, scientists found other such viruses, perhaps twenty in all by the mid-1960s, linked to cancer in a tremendous variety of animal species. There was simian sarcoma virus, believed to cause tumors in monkeys under certain circumstances, mouse sarcoma virus, avian leukosis virus. The virologists and most other biologists naturally believed that it was only a matter of time before they would find the viruses responsible for human cancers.

A matter of time and, of course, money.

Throughout the 1960s and most of the 1970s cancer meant "open sesame" to the federal research vault. Not that any proposal mentioning the word would automatically be funded; but it had become a standing joke among investigators that if you could relate a project to conquering cancer, chances for funding increased manyfold. Weinberg himself says with characteristically blunt simplicity that showing a project's relationship to cancer was "necessary to get money to run your laboratory."

From the mid-1960s through the 1970s, virology was among the best cared for and most widely funded of molecular biology's subspecialties. That the virus was or was not a neat model for gene behavior was a matter for academic debate; finding the cause of cancer was of immediate, passionate public concern. Nothing seemed more plausible than that viruses would prove to be that cause, and that virologists would find the right ones and their mechanisms of action.

Humans' genetic makeup varies by surprisingly little from that of other mammals. It is because the genes of most mammals are so similar, for example, that humans have been able to use insulin isolated from slaughtered pigs and cows; the genes that yield this vital hormone are nearly identical across the species. Further, although viruses can be specific to certain species, often as not a given type will infect a broad range of species. The same virus that causes rabies in dogs causes rabies in squirrels and other rodents and, passed on through a bite, in humans. The bubonic plague bacterium that infects rats can be transmitted by rats' fleas to humans. There had never been found a whole category of infectious agents from which human beings alone among mammals were exempt.

Even more to the point, humans *get* cancer, so it was perfectly logical to assume they contracted it from the same source as other mammals.

Remember that the study of viruses had two distinct, not necessarily related aims: Basic scientists were primarily interested in viruses as a source of pure knowledge, insights into the elemental behavior of genes; their second goal was to find a viral cause of cancer. The second aim provided virtually all the money for the first. One of the great ironies in the search is that the virologists' enormous contribution to cancer research had far more to do with the virus as a model of gene behavior, with what viruses have taught us about basic gene behavior, than it had with discovery of the first human cancer virus; further, many of those who were most critical of the virologists' "academic" absorptions provided the tools without which little more would be known of cancer today than was known in 1978.

But that is way ahead of the story. By the late 1970s, some fifteen years and many millions of dollars down the road and well into the "war on cancer," the virologists had yet to locate a single virus that could be implicated even remotely in human tumors. Their stock was at a low. From about the mid-1970s, their views had been greeted with mounting skepticism by other scientists. Not that they were in disgrace—certainly Weinberg does not speak of that period in such terms—but to hear of it from many virologists then at the National Cancer Institute, where the political winds blow strongest, they were frequently viewed as pursuing phantoms to justify their basic research.

It was becoming increasingly obvious that either (a) There were no human cancer viruses, in which case the virologists had been headed in the wrong direction; or (b) There were such viruses and the virologists had spent millions of dollars without finding them. Either way, the bottom line looked pretty grim.

Perhaps the most persistent of those hunting the elusive human tumor virus was the NCI's own Robert Gallo, whose story is as full of as many twists and ironic turns as any in the cancer war. A colleague in Houston recalled, "Bob put up with years of virtual abuse when people almost claimed he was a charlatan, raising money to look for a cancer virus that plainly did not exist. A lot of his ideas were considered completely off the wall." That slang term for an idea that is, let's say, slightly screwy is a favorite among biologists; and too many off-the-wall ideas can label a scientist as, if not screwy, not to be taken seriously.

It was Gallo who found the first human cancer virus, a cause of one kind of leukemia. But by the time Gallo announced the discovery of human T-cell leukemia virus (HTLV) in 1980, not even he believed that viruses were the direct cause of more than a few human cancers—and those, so far, are rare ones.

Just as frustration was peaking over the failure to locate human cancer viruses, chemical carcinogenesis came into vogue, perhaps coincidentally. During the late 1970s, scientists, environmentalists, and many others scrutinized industrial wastes and chemicals as possible sources of human cancers, and some alarmists proclaimed that the nation was in the middle of a cancer epidemic caused by industrial waste. (That almost certainly is not the case. See page 36 for John Cairns's discussion of cancer epidemiology.)

George Khoury, chief of the NCI's laboratory of molecular virology, noted that there was strong competition for research money between those studying chemical carcinogenesis and the virologists, and the latter suddenly found themselves in leaner times after a decade of relatively easy funding. "People like Bob Weinberg and Mike Bishop," and others persisted in their conviction instead of following the new trend. The perception was that ultimately *either* chemicals *or* viruses were the villains in human cancer, and viruses were looking increasingly dim as the culprits.

And here is the problem weighing on Weinberg as he makes his way across Longfellow Bridge on a bitter winter night. The whole theory of cancer causation was breaking up into competing parts; the unity that gives power to scientific ideas was eroding.

Weinberg considers: There is a transforming principle involved in cancer, a genetically based principle that will make an ordinary cell cancerous. This principle operates when cancer viruses infect chickens, but it operates equally when a chemical carcinogen causes a cell to transform from normal to tumorous. So the principle is not a virus per se, nor a chemical per se. It is the target of either of those. And when a child never known to have been exposed to a carcinogen gets cancer, it is that principle at work. A common thread. A unity underlying apparent diversity.

It was in chemical transformation, Weinberg suddenly realized, that the key to finding this principle lay. It was known that if you cancerously transformed cells in culture with a virus, you could use those cells to transform healthy cells. But was the transforming principle viral? Cellular? In the genes of either? Consider starting with cells transformed by a chemical. It was known that chemical carcinogens mutated genes. Second, the chemical would ultimately be diluted out of the mix in a string of serial transfections: Would the cells continue transforming one another—transformed cell acting on healthy cell, and so on?

Finally, if a sequence of many genes were required to transform a cell, this experiment could not work. The odds of even two genes randomly getting into the cell were astronomical. If this experiment worked it would be because one aberrant gene tripped the cell into cancerous behavior.

Like most pivotal realizations—and Weinberg remembers this as one that changed his life, that shaped his views as a scientist—this one depended for its execution on ideas that had been worked out by hundreds of other scientists in other specialties. Cell biologists and physicians had developed clear descriptions for transformation in a cell, the distinctive biological behavior of the cancerous cell that they called its "phenotype." Bacterial researchers had developed the methods for moving genes from cell to cell, and one classical cell biologist named Michael Wigler at the Cold Spring Harbor Biological Laboratories on Long Island had helped develop methods for carrying out these procedures within the forbidding complexities of mammalian cells. Oncogene discoveries are the greatest current example of synergy or cooperation in scientific research, in which discoveries in one area augment those in another, in which a single discovery by one investigator may owe major credit to the seemingly unrelated work of dozens of others in different fields.

When biologists say they have transformed a cell, do they mean they have given it cancer? Yes and no. They mean they have made cells in a laboratory dish fulfill certain criteria associated with cancer-cell behavior. They assert that the one set of behaviors *in vitro*, in the glass of the laboratory dish, parallels the cancer behaviors *in vivo*, in the living system. And as we'll see, the contention is frequently disputed.

Here is the biological behavior or phenotype of cancerous cells that Weinberg used in 1978 and that is still used as the test for *in vitro* laboratory transformation.

1. Transformed cells are *anchorage independent*. Normal cells must adhere to a surface in order to carry out their biological

activities. In the body this surface is a layer of support tissue through which the cell receives nutriment and instructions on how to behave. In the laboratory this is the surface of a dish. The normal cell needs such a surface; the transformed cell can float freely in a thick liquid nutrient, grow, and multiply.

2. Cancer cells have *reduced serum requirements.* They can be sustained on a level of nutrients that would not allow normal cells to remain alive.

3. Normal cells have *contact inhibition.* They grow with great difficulty in a laboratory dish, and then they grow only one layer deep, ceasing growth when they contact a neighboring cell. Under the microscope they resemble a neatly laid-out cobblestone mosaic. Transformed cells grow in jumbled bunches, stacking atop one another like a pile of cobblestones erupting in midpattern along a cobblestone street. This would turn out to be the most important feature of transformed cells in identifying them in the laboratory (see Figure 2).

A colony of normal mammalian cells growing in a dish would show up as a pale, filmy cast the color of whatever dye or other chemical stained them, a monolayer, one cell thick. But look at a dish containing transformed cells and you can plainly see small, dark-colored spots, dark stars within the pale field, marking the focus of each packed colony of cancer cells. These dense spots are called

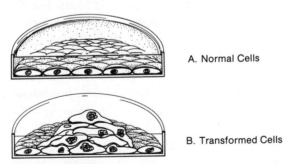

A. Normal Cells

B. Transformed Cells

Figure 2. Animal cells ordinarily grow only one layer deep in a cell culture because they have "contact inhibition," their growth ceasing as soon as they touch another cell. Transformed cells lose that inhibition and grow in jumbles.

foci (plural of focus, and pronounced FO-si). Searching for them, counting them, and recording their number would consume much of the time in Weinberg's laboratory for several years to come.

Weinberg's plan was to chemically transform mouse cells with a carcinogen called methylcholanthrene. He would then remove the genes (that is, the DNA alone) from the transformed cells and add them to a fresh batch of mouse cells, looking for further transformation. Naturally, some of the carcinogen might carry over and be cited as the real cause of the "cancer" in the new dishes. But if he kept going, serially transferring transformed cells' genes from dish to dish, the chemical would plainly be diluted out of the mix. If the transformation continued unabated, then the chemical clearly was only the agent, the triggering device, and there was a target which, once transformed, induced transformation in each successive transfer. No virus would be present, and since the target of chemical carcinogens was known to be the genes, then this transforming principle in this case would be demonstrated to reside within one altered gene of the original mouse cells.

From the moment he thought of it, Weinberg was "utterly convinced" it would work. Few others were. Others had tried somewhat similar experiments aimed at proving the same thing with no results, wasting months of time and money in searches for transformed colonies that were never found. In fact, a researcher had just reported in the prestigious journal *Cell* that he had succeeded with virtually the same experiment Weinberg was about to try, but the article had to be retracted when the researcher's findings were thrown into disrepute, and Michael Wigler recalled that he and others turned sharply away from that avenue of inquiry because it was tainted by scandal.

But Weinberg, through some twist of fate, had missed the article. On the night he conceived his scheme for finding the transforming principle, he was unaware anyone had laid claim to it, and by the time he learned that earlier results had been published but discredited, he was far down the road and doubly determined that his own results would be utterly beyond reproach.

He and graduate student Mitch Goldfarb spent weeks chemically transforming mouse cells, removing the DNA, putting it in normal-mouse-cell cultures, staring at the pale dishes for the dark stars that

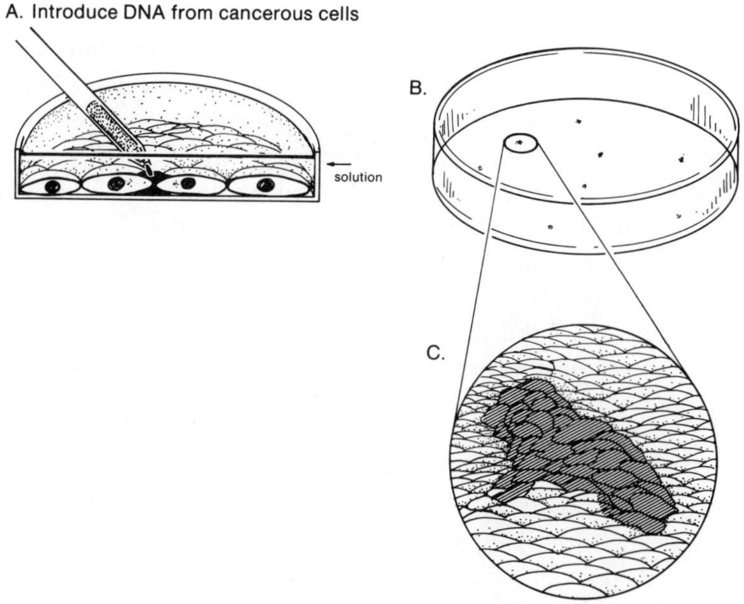

A. Introduce DNA from cancerous cells

solution

B.

C.

Figure 3. *The biological properties of transformed cells can be used to show that the "transforming principle" resides in the DNA. A: The fragmented DNA of transformed cells is introduced into a culture of normal mouse cells. B: Some cells taking up the DNA are themselves transformed, losing their contact inhibition and growing in a pile. C: When placed in a petri dish, the transformed colonies appear as tiny dark stars against the background monolayer of normal cells.*

would tell them new transformation had occurred (see Figure 3). The search in fact was far more difficult than just described. In culture, cells of the type Weinberg was using will spontaneously transform now and then; therefore, even without a carcinogen, a culture of these mouse cells will show a background of transformed dark stars, a kind of background noise in the pale monolayer. When cells were chemically transformed, the number of foci soared well beyond this background. The problem for Weinberg and Goldfarb was to distinguish between truly transformed colonies and those containing only background eruptions, and that was in itself a formidable challenge, especially in the climate of doubt and distrust that now existed.

The weeks became months. At several points, Goldfarb counted what both he and Weinberg believed were "credible foci," but they neither saw enough nor were the properties sufficiently demonstrable for Weinberg, who has a reputation for caution and thoroughness, to leap into print. Now it was time for Goldfarb to finish his doctoral thesis and graduate. They had tried every technique they could think of for introducing the chemically transformed DNA into fresh mouse cells and reading the results, with no real luck.

Goldfarb moved on to new research as a postdoctoral fellow in the laboratory of Michael Wigler, the same Wigler who had done the major groundwork indicating that it would be possible to transfect genes in difficult-to-use mammal cells, and who would become a major competitor of Weinberg's in the oncogene race.

That Weinberg persisted—as did Wigler and Bishop and a handful of others—may not seem unusual, but other scientists find it remarkable. Weinberg was now in his late thirties; he had tenure at MIT and a good working relationship in his laboratory, but despite a reputation for doing good science, he had not made a name for himself. It was a dangerous time to be looking for funds and more funds to chase down what was very likely a blind alley.

Chiaho Shih, a new graduate student, took over Goldfarb's work when Goldfarb left. More months went by, during which Shih developed his own technique for "scoring" foci, a somewhat more objective method of reading the foci for transformations that might occur above the background. This promised to be a fruitful method for determining results, but it still was somewhat subjective—that is, the results could be influenced by what the investigator wanted to see.

To make sure that he and Shih would not see what they desperately wanted to see rather than what had grown in the laboratory dishes, Weinberg took the precaution of having Shih read the foci "blind." That is, Weinberg coded the dozens of dishes involved in each experiment so that only he knew which ones ought to contain the "transforming principle" among the DNA and which ones were controls—parallel mouse-cell cultures, one treated with chemically transformed DNA, one with normal.

More than a year after Weinberg's brainstorm, the results came in. He was finally confronted with solid evidence that transformation was occurring just as he had believed—by action of genes and genes alone. Over and over again, Shih found transformation, cancerous cell behavior, where it should have been, traceable in a long unbroken course down descendant colonies of cells that had lost their growth controls just by inheriting that damaged gene, the oncogene. Look: no chemical present, no virus; just genes. An altered gene introduced into normal cells caused them to become cancerous, altering their genes so that future generations of cells would also be cancerous.

Sophisticated as modern biology is in concept, and even though it employs some complex machinery, most experiments come down to observation by a scientist with the naked eye. These experiments were no exception, and although Weinberg was not challenged on the accuracy of his readings, it became plain that there were many doubters in the science community who believed, and offered good reasons for believing, that what had been at long last successfully carried out in glass dishes was not the same as what was going on in the cancer-stricken human.

Weinberg was asked later if his belief that he could prove cancer to be inducible purely by this gene transfer had been considered "off the wall."

"Not off the wall, no," he recalled. Summer now, several summers later, a time when white-sailed boats by the dozens blew up and down the Charles River: "Obscure. The idea was considered interesting but obscure, something that might prove intellectually interesting but would have no application whatever to human cancer."

In science, the finder of an answer becomes a target; the bigger the prospective answer, the bigger the target, and that is an important part of the scientific process. The discoverer expects challenge on every major issue and technique and on the reading of results that led to his conclusion. That's an important way to weed error and "artifact" out of science. Weinberg got his challenge, although he says the questions were no more than he'd bargained for.

The summer of the first successful transfection experiments, 1979, Weinberg went to a Gordon conference in New Hampshire, excited to be able to report to colleagues what he and Shih were readying for publication. The Gordon conferences, several dozen of them held every summer in virtually all branches of science, are among the most prestigious in the nation. The settings are usually rural New England prep schools closed for the summer. Participants attend by invitation only. They spend mornings and evenings for a week talking science, afternoons hiking, boating, and playing volleyball, softball, and basketball, then the late evenings quaffing great quantities of beer, talking on into the wee hours, many until dawn. The atmosphere is heady, say those who have attended; there, especially during the long nights, science is at its best: open, informal, no holds barred.

Weinberg was "politely" received at the Gordon conference, but if they expected universal acceptance of their findings, he did not get it. Challenges to the experiments and to subsequent experiments by other researchers seeking to prove related ideas would continue for many years, and some would come from leaders in cancer biology.

All the challenges might be summarized roughly this way:

The results were equivocal; they did not prove that a gene or genes alone could transform a normal cell. Reason: Weinberg and Shih had not started with normal cells. Rather, they had used a line of mouse connective-tissue cells bred by Howard Green, then an MIT scientist and now chairman of physiology at Harvard Medical School. Using mice provided by the National Institutes of Health, Green bred a cell line for research purposes that had a quality mammalian cells normally lack: These cells would grow on and on, not stopping after about five divisions. Frequently referred to as "immortalized," they already imitated much of the behavior of cancer cells. This cell line, NIH3t3, already well known to researchers, would become even better known in the controversy over the experiments.

Green had bred NIH3t3 cells specifically so they would be easier to grow than ordinary cells; but maybe they were easier to grow because they were halfway down the road toward cancer, needing only a nudge to push them over.

Perhaps, therefore, what Weinberg and Shih had found was simply a gene that removes contact inhibition, allowing the cells to grow in a jumble, and maybe that was the last remaining transformed behavior the cell line still lacked.

Had the experimenters achieved success with ordinary mouse cells, connective tissue of the same type as the NIH3t3 cells? They had not.

More seriously, other critics thought that the so-called oncogenes were actually oddities of the laboratory that would in certain ways mimic the behavior going on in "real" cancer but that were not causes of such behavior. In laboratory dishes, under the direction of onco-genes, cells might grow wildly into a tumorlike mass, but that did not prove that cancerous tumors grew under such aberrant direction in the human body.

Scientists are forever trying to imitate the world at large in their laboratories, to derive true analogies of how diseases develop or life processes are carried out, and the history of science is full of ex-amples of false appearances, of evidence that seems to prove a theory only to be ultimately uncovered as an accident of the laboratory.

Such false appearances are called artifacts by scientists. In the physical sciences artifact has virtually the opposite meaning it has in common usage. Far from being a "true relic," artifact implies artifice or mirage, an accident that is not recognized by the experi-menter. The most serious criticism one scientific investigator can level at another, short of questioning the researcher's integrity, is to suggest that key findings are artifactual.

What some of the challengers over the years suggested was that the NIH3t3 cell line itself was an artifact, and it fit some of their ideas of an artifact to a T: The results reported might be due to the experi-mental system, not nature's behavior. The results tell us how some odd cells behave in Bob Weinberg's lab, not how cells behave in the tumor of a human body, or even of a mouse's normal connective tissue.

Finally, what is cancer? Is it simply an uncontrolled proliferation of cells, a transformation of cells? Isn't *malignancy* characterized by invasion of *other* tissues by cancer cells, and *metastasis* by the travel of colonies of cancer cells to distant sites in the body?

Weinberg has unwaveringly believed that each of these challenges would be met. Most have been. Some are still debated. "One has to be a fanatic," he said, "to keep at something when you're sure you're right, until you prove it."

They were a small group of scientists, related by the mutual con-viction that oncogenes held the secret to human cancer. Often they sharply disagreed on other matters, but such is typical of the breed. How they would respond to these challenges formed the basis of most of their work over the following years—and led to some of the more important discoveries about the molecular–genetic basis of cancer. Those later discoveries are understandable only in a wider context, at a later time in the story.

But what had begun with the work of Bishop and Varmus, Ames, Wigler, and, in a major way, Weinberg became a broad range of discoveries, far more important than even they believed was so close at hand. Virology, cytology, classical genetics—each a close, tight subspecialty, each with its own relationship to molecular biology— were being fused to emerge in the 1980s as the science of molecular genetics. The single force that energized this fusion was the search for the cause of cancer. The process of finding that cause: the challenge and counterchallenge, the never-ending skepticism, of science.

In late 1982, for example, Weinberg succeeded in proving he could transform *normal* mouse cells with oncogenes, meeting what most considered to be the most serious of the challenges summarized. Yet by the summer of 1984, more than a year after those results were obtained, they were still hotly disputed by some of the best among Weinberg's colleagues.

Chemical transformation with methylcholanthrene, it eventually was learned, activated a single oncogene in the original mouse cell. Two scientists in Weinberg's lab, whose work will be explored in detail later, discovered that the key to transforming *normal* mouse cells requires activating two oncogenes—not just any two, but the right two. In other words, one oncogene might transform an already established or immortalized cell line like NIH3t3, but just two would transform even normal mouse cells.

These results were exciting, because one can imagine a scenario in which one oncogene "immortalizes" the cell line so it will keep growing and dividing, as the NIH3t3 line already did; when the second oncogene "turns on," or goes into action, it completes the transformation. It is a pretty picture, neat and simple, and it fits the decades-old belief that cancer is a multistep process. But in the summer of 1984 could be heard this challenge, so similar in kind to those of 1979: "So you put two genes together and you get transformation, where one alone would not work. Well, maybe one oncogene shakes the cell up and two shake it up a hell of a lot, so over it goes [into cancer]. Is that the way cancer works outside the laboratory dish?"

The man saying that is Michael Wigler, mammalian gene wizard, one of those whose work established the whole oncogene theory of cancer causation. In science the same questions often circle and circle back again, long after they had seemed answered, whirling back in only slightly altered form. And now the deadly artifact wheeled by again: Have you imitated nature or falsified it? Is this Reality or illusion?

But there are few who still doubt the findings of 1979: Cancer is caused by the action of one or more oncogenes, the aberrant genetic elements deep within the cell, the regions of the chemical DNA that determine the inherited characteristics, the growth and development, of all life on earth.

As will be seen, Weinberg is convinced that this two-oncogene synergy will prove a major discovery along the road to finding cancer's pathway. Real cancer. Human cancer. In July of 1984 he would say, in his clearly enunciated, firm yet low voice: "I have a picture in my mind of how cancer works—a model, if you will, that shows each step, from the beginning through metastasis."

Metastasis: the invasion of distant parts of the body by tumor cells, the system-wide form of cancer that is most deadly. Virtually every cancer doctor says something like this: You can show me cells proliferating in a dish ad nauseam. Show me how one of these cells goes off and colonizes tissues at a distant site, creating microtumors all over the body. Show me that, or don't say you're showing me cancer. Metastasis is the end of the story.

"Someone in my lab is working right now on finding a gene or genes which I believe causes metastasis," Weinberg said. "Ask me in two months and I believe he will have found the answer. In my mind, I am utterly convinced that it works this way."

2

Open Desert

At least this much now seems virtually certain: Cancer is a disease of the genes, of the genetic message center inside of each cell in the body. That doesn't mean it's necessarily passed on from one generation to the next, although in some cases a predisposition to cancer may be inherited. The more usual causal pathway, which doctors call the etiology, seems to involve damage to genes of the living cell well after birth. The first problem in trying to understand cancer at this most basic level is to get some sense of proportion, a consistent idea of the shape and scale of things in a submicroscopic world beyond the reach of vision. A few of the elements of molecular genetics are visible beneath the light microscope—human cells, the chromosomes that DNA is packed into in higher animals—but they are planet-sized on the scale of single genes and DNA components, and for that reason these latter must always be renderings, sketches, schematic no matter how lifelike we intend them to be (see Figure 4).

DNA—deoxyriboneucleic acid—was earlier referred to as the chemical molecule that holds the entire code for living things on earth. Chromosomes are packages of DNA and packing material; genes are physically nothing but specific regions along a DNA molecule. Think of computer punch tape, a long paper ribbon whose perforations are coded symbols. DNA represents a collection of such symbols,

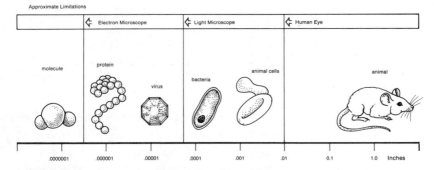

Figure 4. *Living things cover an enormous spectrum of sizes. Cells are on a size order beginning just below the visible—below one-hundredth of an inch on the chart. The light microscope reveals objects down to about one ten-thousandth of an inch. Electron micrographs offer depictions of matter analogous to visual renderings down to just under one-millionth of an inch. Below that limit is the wholly invisible world of molecules, whose shapes and dimensions are inferred experimentally.*

and a gene represents a particular group of symbols within such a collection.

But talk of genes and the DNA code units making them up and we're in a world of molecules some of whose dimensions are on the same scale as wavelengths of light. Molecules are composed of atoms, which in turn are more than 99.9 percent empty space. In other words, on this scale when light reflects or is absorbed it does not lend form the way it does for objects in the visible world, even in the world visible under the light microscope. This is a level at which objects or particles devour light waves—absorb them—and are excited into vibrations, into changes in shape and ultimately identity by the light's energy, or by energy from x-rays or electricity or even other molecules. So we begin in a quandary: We have to *imagine* seeing the things in this world in order to understand them in human terms, knowing that by this very association we are losing precision in their definition.

Driving alone across the country there's a lot of time for the imagination to play. The variety of the countryside, open and flat, mountainous, desert; the tightness and angularity of the city; the geometry of farmland; night and day—all these encourage a lot of different patterns of thinking, particular and vivid, then abstract. My first step, from the southeastern corner of Phoenix to Tucson, is about one hundred miles of hot, flat desert, the scrubland of the often beautiful Sonoran; it leaves a great deal of room for the imagination.

Imagine for openers that we are going to make visible and give familiar shapes to these elemental parts of life systems. Like modern sculptors we are constructing huge works in various colors, and they move according to our design. Imagine now we are choreographers in a theater designed for such works, that we will make them sway, coil, unbend, combine, dance to whatever rhythms we provide. We are going to create a drama to beggar the imagination. There's just one catch (there always is): This entire effort at shaping models in our minds is aimed at imitating nature as closely as possible, as faithfully as our best intellectual and physical efforts can achieve. Imagine we are playing nature—that we are scientists.

*   *   *

In this theater of the mind, we have trained a spotlight on a single human cell.* The only thing that's important about it is its scale in relation to some of the components deep inside it. In reality the cell is about one hundred microns across—not that far below the visible range; ten cells laid side by side would stretch a millimeter, around one-fiftieth of an inch. Under the spotlight the cell looks like a transparent bag of clear jelly about the size of a basketball, within which are suspended various subunits. The bag now swells, expands in size until it fills the whole of the darkened theater, continues to swell until it fills our whole perception. Its curved surface becomes as large as a domed stadium—say Houston's Astrodome, since I'm headed that way. Now we are at the entrance of the Astrodome; the far wall is two hundred yards away. From here the cell's nucleus, its command center, is a sphere within the sphere, covering the whole of

---

* The major scientific concepts involved in cancer research, as I review them in this mind-theater, will be set off by three asterisks at the beginning and end of the passages. Follow them step by step or return to them later; they are clearly identified in the index.

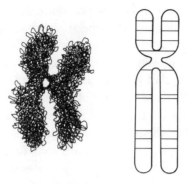

Figure 5. Chromosomes are long strands of DNA gathered like wool on a skein, as shown on the left. When chemically stained for viewing under the light microscope, chromosomes show distinctive banding patterns which scientists use in schematic drawings, as shown on the right, to help identify chromosomes and to mark locations of particular genes.

the infield. Move inward, let the swelling form expand still further, and imagine we are looking, close up, at this nucleus, now swollen as large as the entire Astrodome itself. The nucleus will have to swell larger for us to make out what's inside it.

Throughout the Astrodome-sized clear ball of nucleus, you can just about make out, when the light strikes your mind in the right way, the fine filament running throughout. Although it is so thin you can barely see it, the filament is very long: It runs, twists, turns everywhere in the clear nucleus. The filament is a molecule of DNA, what Francis Crick called the brain of the cell.

This model is unrealistic in one sense. The DNA of a bacterial cell might look like this; but in the cells of humans and other more complex organisms (see Figure 5), the DNA is broken up into long pieces that are coiled and twisted around their packing material, like yarn on a skein, into the shapes called chromosomes. But for now we can imagine the DNA has been stretched out and stuck together into a single molecule. That molecule contains the entire genetic inheritance of the organism whose cell it is within. It is a molecule composed of many thousands of smaller units, and those units contain all the information needed to build a human being or a mouse, an eagle or a worm, depending on the ordering of the molecule's subunits. It contains enough information not only to build the physical creature but to maintain the operation of all its cells. In this computer punch tape each base unit represents a code letter; in that respect it is conceptually very simple, but here simplicity leaves us.

Not surprisingly, it takes a library's worth of information to build a baby inside its mother's womb, out of materials shipped in through the umbilical cord. One message unit of this DNA is so small that it would take twenty billion units laid side by side to stretch six feet—yet there are so many message units that six feet is about the actual length of the DNA tightly coiled inside each cell of a human body. Put another way, if these message units were one-half-inch long, the chain would stretch more than 15,000 miles, halfway around the world.

Genes, the units of inheritance now so strongly implicated in cancer, each consist of anywhere from a thousand to forty thousand of these base message units, so at one-half inch per unit, one gene would be a string of instructions anywhere from forty feet to a mile long. That enormous variation also offers a clue to why understanding a particular gene's structure and function is so difficult.

For future reference it will be important to understand the shape as well as the scale of DNA, because a great deal of the way it works relates to that shape; to anyone interested in design this molecule, in fact, is a masterpiece. But when we try to visualize DNA, we are playing another mind game: We are creating a gaudy representation to explain something that really has no "look" to it at all.

In the early 1950s the leading biochemists in the world were in a tense race to see who would be first to determine the shape of DNA, a determination that would, it was correctly believed, lead to an understanding of its function. James Watson and Francis Crick did it in 1953 and got the Nobel Prize for their efforts. They studied the patterns x-rays made as they shot through and bounced off the molecule, mixed in their knowledge of the angles and distances between atoms in certain kinds of molecules, squeezed it all through the prism of genius, and came up with a model not much different from the one I'm preparing to bang together. (Theirs was assembled from

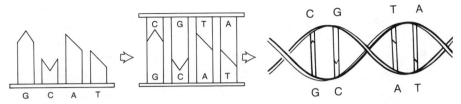

Figure 6. Left: *The genetic code is carried in four bases whose abbreviations (A,T,C,G) are like letters in a special alphabet. Although all four are different sizes (center), base pairs A-T and G-C form congruent steps that are joined into a ladderlike structure by external backbones, then twisted, as on the right, into the double helix of the DNA molecule.*

rods and sheet metal by the metal shop at Cambridge University in England.)

DNA is often referred to as a "double helix" (the title of Watson's memoir of the period). That is, it is formed of two long strands of "bases" that have been linked together and then given a twist, like a spiral staircase. The molecular message units referred to earlier—the individual symbols punched in the computer tape—are, chemically speaking, four bases named adenine, guanine, cytosine, and thymine. Shorthand: A, G, C, T. Each of these represents a letter in DNA language, but the language can be saved for later.

To build a model of DNA, think of each of the four bases as a piece of plywood, its shape somewhat irregular and not exactly like any of the other three. But because the shapes are complementary, base A always naturally binds to base T, and base C always adjoins base G. The bases bind edge to edge. That's significant, because thus joined, each base-pair forms a neat rectangle, and the AT rectangle is congruent with the GC rectangle (see Figure 6). Thus, although no two bases are the same shape, that becomes irrelevant to the carpentry: AT is the same shape as GC. Each is one step in the ladder. For the sides, hammer a support structure to link the steps together at the outsides and bang it all together into a ladder. Twist the ladder at each end in opposite directions and you approximate a spiral staircase, a double helix.

Densely packed together so only one-half inch separates each step of the model, the spiral staircase approximating the DNA region for one long gene would run about a mile; for a short one, forty feet. The human body contains about 100,000 genes, some long, some short, strung together with mysterious regions of DNA that apparently code for nothing.

The purpose of this double-helical model, in life-systems terms, is to provide information; conceptually, this is fairly simple. Take that double helix and strip it in half, unzip it so you've pulled apart the ladder at the steps where the base pairs join. Now you can read along one edge and you might see this base sequence:

C–G–G–C–A–G–C–C–A

This will later turn out to be a particularly interesting base sequence, but for now, I might have invented it for an imaginary gene. Remembering that the base units zip up complementarily, with A bonding only to T and G only to C, by reading the above base sequence you would know that opposite it when the DNA is twined in its double helix you would read this:

G–C–C–G–T–C–G–G–T

But let's concentrate on the first sequence and assume it defines a portion of a gene. The first step in every genetic activity, no matter how complex, lies within the DNA molecule. First, a gene "switches on," becomes active and able to be interpreted, or "read." Then, in a long and complex process (see pp. 40–41), its instructions are followed in a chain of molecular events. The instructions depend simply on the order of the bases being read, just as letters of the alphabet code for words, then sentences. The gene is an actual template; alongside the gene region a long, single-chain molecule will form, "picking up" the instructions of the gene in its own order of bases.

What is the end of the whole process? For *what* are these genes coding? For proteins. True, the genes also must code for many of the intermediary molecules in the production line, but the end product of gene activation is a protein, one gene being defined as the amount of coding needed to direct production of one protein. We are creatures made of protein and other chemicals made by those proteins. Proteins are the major structural building blocks of each cell.

They are responsible for the growth and repair of the body. Special kinds of proteins—enzymes—regulate virtually every chemical action within the cell, and other specialized proteins—hormones—communicate large-scale messages from one part of the body to another. Enzymes carry out the reactions that cause a cell to grow and divide into two new "daughter" cells, and other enzymes control those reactions.

Loss of growth, of course, is the most commonly cited feature of cancer. A normal cell grows and divides a few times, lives its span of anywhere from hours to an adult lifetime, depending on its type, and then it dies. The cancer cell grows and divides, grows and divides, on and on, until a single misdirected cell becomes a tumor colony of identical cells—each under the irregular growth control of the same gene or genes. Some cells might revert to normal, their cancer-genes' instructions having perhaps been corrected. But on balance a tumor might continue to grow because enough cells are still growing and dividing that the net effect is a steady proliferation. That at least is what is currently meant by oncogenes: genes with fouled instructions, or normal genes whose instructions to produce growth enzymes are being read when they should not be.

But this model is so abstract! A visualizing beyond direct visual confirmation. It is general human nature to want to see before believing; for scientists, especially molecular biologists, it is an obsession. "I wanted to *see* something," said MIT's David Baltimore, describing what was goading him onward on the day when as an undergraduate he talked his way into a Cold Spring Harbor laboratory to see under a microscope the microorganisms he had only heard lectured about.

Yet, years later, what Baltimore eventually "saw" that won him the Nobel Prize was another of those genetic elements turning in a world far below the microscopic, far below seeing; his discovery would prove a vital milestone on the road to explaining cancer, but one whose function will only become clear later. And Watson and Crick, who more than any other scientists set modern biology on its course in 1953, are always referred to as having "elucidated the shape of DNA," light having now become a metaphor. But just when it would be tempting to limit the real world to what can be seen and touched, we have to admit that the real world begins within those 99.9

percent-empty-space atoms, and the real world has cancer; where it originates we hope to discover.

* * *

"I keep thinking how strange it is to be reading these symptoms in my textbook, studying for finals, and I recognize my own symptoms." Belinda Mims, sitting on a hospital bed, says this with laughter in her voice, a laughter her mother tries to share, cannot quite, but acknowledges with an admiring nod. "I'm not really worried. I haven't been all along. I'm going to make it."

Mims, twenty-one years old, a fourth-year pharmacy student at the University of Arizona in Tucson, found a lump in her neck in mid-April 1984. It didn't go away. Later she developed the flulike symptoms often associated with Hodgkin's disease, but by then it was already suspected. She showed the lump to her roommate, a medical student, and the roommate took Belinda to one of her own medical professors. That path led to Dr. Hugo Villar, surgeon. Chest x-rays showed Mims had multiple tumors in her chest cavity, but none below the rib cage—a distinction that is important in "staging" Hodgkin's: the farther the tumors have spread, the graver the illness. A biopsy confirmed the tumors and the extent of their spread through her system.

Hodgkin's disease is a form of lymphoma—cancer of the lymphocytes found in lymph fluid and other cells. Lymph is part of a circulatory system that runs parallel to the bloodstream. Its job is to cleanse cells and tissues of wastes, dumping them into the bloodstream for removal. The lymph nodes, which represent junctures where several ducts come together and concentrate their wastes, are likely points for infection, and swellings in such nodes usually indicate nothing more serious than infection. But the nodes also offer likely latch points for the traveling microtumors called metastases.

Hodgkin's disease has virtually always metastasized by the time it is found; for that reason it used to be almost uniformly fatal. The recent history of treatment of this disease is one of the true bright spots in the cancer story, with survival rates now running very high, better than 50 percent, and even higher than that for young people.

In the morning, Mims will have her spleen removed, because the spleen, with a high concentration of lymphocyte cells, is a likely site for metastasis. She anticipates living a relatively normal life without it, without further recurrence of the disease. Her optimism is infectious. Sitting on her bed here at the Arizona Cancer Center, legs crossed, she looks and sounds like a coed chatting with friends.

She took her final examination in pharmacology early this afternoon, her last of the term. She has another year to go in the five-year program at the University of Arizona and plans to finish on time. "Nothing was going to interfere with finals," she says, but the cancer finally did. She had to take makeup exams because of the timing of her biopsy, but she thinks she did better than usual because she used the medical school's nearby extensive library to prepare. The exam she had been talking about, surprising her as her textbook mirrored her life, was on diseases, and the section on cancers included Hodgkin's.

It can be frustrating, whether student, patient, or writer, to try to pin down the cure rates for these cancers, and Hodgkin's is no exception, but not because anyone is trying to fudge figures. Part of the problem is that the outlook for patients can be radically different depending on how they are categorized. Over the years, epidemiologists, specialists in the spread of disease, have profiled virtually every cancer by every means at their disposal: What is the survival rate for patients of each age group, of each stage in the cancer's progress? What are the other risk factors particular to that disease? To say that Mims has a particular chance of being cured without knowing the risk factors is impossible. Villar, her surgeon, of course does know them, and he says her odds for complete recovery are good.

Meanwhile, Belinda remains the cheerful bulwark of her family, mother Diane says, in what has been a very tough year for mother, father, and only child. Belinda was born in Tucson, but the family now lives in Mississippi, where Wayne Mims works for Georgia Pacific. Six months earlier, his mother had died of kidney cancer. Belinda couldn't make it home then. "I felt bad about it," she says. But then when her own cancer was diagnosed she told her mother to stay home until it was almost time for her surgery. Diane recalls that after his mother's death, Wayne had consoled himself that, dying at age seventy-two, she had lived a full life. No such consolation was available when they learned Belinda had Hodgkin's. And in between those two nadirs, Wayne Mims was diagnosed as having lupus, an arthritis-like disease, a diagnosis later changed to rheuma-toid arthritis.

Hodgkin's is one of the few cancers that has what doctors call a "dual profile." If you stand back far enough to generalize about *all* cancers, without discrimination of type, they are diseases of older people; one's chances of getting some form of cancer increase markedly after age fifty. Cancers that zero in on young people are fewer in number, much rarer in occurrence, and now are generally the more curable, thanks to remarkable progress in chemotherapy.

Cancers with dual profiles strike two different age groups. Hodgkin's first strikes young people, just about Belinda's age, usually is not seen in adults in their mid-twenties through their forties, then affect those middle-aged and older. Mims also exemplifies another major feature of the profile of young Hodgkin's victims: She is the only child of a relatively well-to-do family. This may be one of the stranger correlations in the pattern of a cancer's occurrence, but it is far from the only strange one, as I would soon learn.

Concerning the unusual Hodgkin's profile, doctors have speculated that relatively well-off only children are probably more protected from dirt and germs than children with brothers and sisters and/or those from poorer families. The unintended consequence could be that the only child's unbattered immune system does not develop fully with-out the school of hard knocks that is the ordinary child's environ-ment. But this is pure speculation. At best, virtually every conversation about cancer has to be doused with perhapses and maybes, and most of the general conclusions about causes are highly speculative.

Maybe that is another reason for the excitement over research findings these days: Even if unproven in the strictest scientific sense, even if scattershot with their own maybes and supposes, the curves on charts scored with error bars, discussions of oncogenes are at least beyond the merely speculative. Oncogenes exist; now they have been found in human tumors, and even more certain lines have been drawn between their actions and the development of tumors.

Down the hall from Mims, Bob Delp and his wife, Vaughn, have just finished talking to Villar about Bob's scheduled spleen removal. He is fifty-two but looks younger, an accomplishment considering that he carried a twenty-pound Hodgkin's tumor inside him until six months ago, when Villar removed it. Now he has been on chemotherapy and radiation, and Villar is very hopeful of his long-term prospects. The Delps have to drive two hundred miles each way from their home in Prescott, north of Phoenix, for treatment, but he considers that a small price to pay.

With vague symptoms of tiredness but no complaints of pain, Delp had begun his long journey to this point in his life, as most cancer patients do, by seeing a local doctor. The doctor referred him to a nearby small hospital, which sent Delp's biopsy off to New Mexico for a pathology report. The pathologist insisted the mass was a fibrous, benign lesion—that was the good news. He also insisted that the twenty-pound tumor could not be removed. "I couldn't figure out what they were all so happy about," Delp says with exasperation. "The doctors come into my room after the biopsy with a bottle of champagne so I can celebrate the fact my tumor wasn't malignant, then tell me I'm going to have to carry it around inside me for the rest of my life."

Luckily, Delp's personal physician, whom he had seen first, was suspicious of the results and sent him to the University of Arizona, which has a specialized cancer center. Delp says he may be one of the few people almost grateful to learn he had a malignant tumor, because when Villar diagnosed it he simultaneously told Delp that it could be removed.

Villar first suspected a malignant tumor because he detected a second pulsebeat under Delp's breastbone, the sign of a tumor's artery supplying blood to the lesion. If the physician fails to detect such a pulsebeat, Hodgkin's can be very difficult to diagnose, because usually only 1 percent of the cells in the tumor are malignant. That is, although all the cells have descended from that first misregulated cell, most of the cells at some point correct themselves—they "terminally divide," stop growing. Enough continue along the erroneous path for the tumor to keep growing and invading, but because the cancerous cells are hidden in a background mass of benign tissue, it is easy to get a false finding that the tumor is benign, a so-called false negative. It becomes even easier to get a misdiagnosis, Villar says, because most people begin the route to cancer treatment at the family physician's and never meet some of the other doctors in the network. As in Delp's case, some of those doctors may have virtually no knowledge of one another's thinking on a particular case they are all working on. Delp never even met the New Mexico pathologist who sent back the reading on the tumor.

That is the idea of a cancer center: to put all the experts together under one roof, where they can talk to one another, attend the same clinical conferences, team up to treat a given case. So, Villar points out, a major part of admitting any new patient to the center is putting together a team consisting of surgeon, chemotherapist, perhaps radiologist and social worker, all of whom are expected to correlate both their observations and their treatment. Arizona's is a small cancer center compared with the giants in the field, but it is well respected. Except for the hospital end of the center, which is a part of the university hospital, the center really consists of a series of prefab buildings out back of the fortresslike hospital–medical college that dominates its Tucson neighborhood. Money has since been granted for a permanent structure for the cancer center, but now as your footsteps resound with the hollow clunk of a wooden floor suspended on air, the cancer center as idea comes through loud and clear. It is in many ways the brainchild of Dr. Sydney Salmon, an internationally recognized myeloma expert, who heads the team of doctors and nurses specializing in cancer treatment and research.

Some of the people who work here are basic researchers, as you'd find in any university—like Robert Trent, a Ph.D. scientist whose name appears in collaboration with the likes of Michael Bishop, Robert Weinberg, and others doing oncogene research. Between this basic research and medical treatment, a great deal of clinical research also goes on here; that is, research into treatment, aimed at finding more successful combinations of drugs, better ways of doing surgery, of detecting cancer earlier, or of preventing it from occurring in the first place.

One researcher here is carrying out a major study on possible cancer-prevention benefits of beta-carotene, the vitamin A precursor that gives carrots their orange color; the value of this and other nutrients is being touted everywhere from here to the National Cancer Institute, which is now pushing the "cancer diet" very hard as a means of prevention.

But if the idea of a cancer center evokes innovation and experiment, you cannot forget for long that you are in a hospital. Dr. Stephen Jones, the center's chief of staff, says at the outset of our conversation on the missions of the center: "We do research, but understand one thing: We treat sick people here, people sick with cancer. Everything we do, everything, is very much related to that idea."

A point well taken, but there seemed to me a hint of challenge in the comment, a suggestion that there might be contention between the doctor in the clinic and the researcher in the lab. Later, farther down the road, such contention would become obvious. From time to time the basic researchers and the doctors, often in collaboration, are, maybe as often, at loggerheads: over funding, over point of view, over what it is we mean when we say "cancer." *We see cancer as it walks in the door. We treat sick people here.*

And those who treat cancer themselves represent an enormous spectrum of outlook between cheerful optimism and dark skepticism. Villar, for example, believes both Mims and Delp have excellent prospects, but for him theirs are bright spots in an otherwise dark terrain. He is one of many physicians and researchers who believe there may have been little if any change in survival rates for cancers, other than for a few like Hodgkin's—so rare compared to lung, breast, colon, and other cancers that are major killers.

Is cancer the disease simple? It is visible; a tumor can be spotted, if not by x-ray then by biopsy. All the vagaries of the microworld are absent: You feel, you operate, you see. As the patient, you survive or you do not. Simple. Except that a whole new range of doubts enters, and these doubts are as frustrating as the impossibility of seeing molecules tumble.

"We have made people more conscious of cancer," says Villar, in his office a dozen yards from the hospital rooms. "Take breast cancer. We have impressed on everyone the importance of early detection, of self-examinations, of physical checkups. For that reason, we are certainly seeing cancer at earlier stages than we used to."

He leans forward, a tall, white-haired man with the Spanish accent of his native Chile. Now he points out the difficulties in trying to assess what is called "the five-year survival rate." Epidemiologists, surveying not one cancer but a whole nation's cancers over many years, must have a variety of ways of judging cures, survival under various treatment regimens. They use five years as the measure of survival of most cancers. If you are alive five years after your last remission in cancer, you have for statistical purposes survived. If the five-year survival rate goes up, epidemiologists say *the* survival rate has gone up. That doesn't seem like a long period to use as final measure, but consider that if a new drug is used to treat cancer, the five-year rate means it will take that long to get a reading on its long-term effectiveness. Now five years can seem like an eternity.

What is bothering Villar bothers many cancer physicians: "Let's assume for the sake of argument that we have not improved a woman's chances of surviving breast cancer one iota. This is purely hypothetical, but let's say that breast cancer takes nine years to grow, develop, and spread, and then it kills, kills most of its victims, and that's the way it's always been. In the past, we would see all our patients entering our offices for the first time in year seven of their cancers. We would treat them for two years, and they would die. So the five-year survival rate would be very low.

"Now we are getting women to detect their cancers early—we see them in year two. We treat them, they live out what is now seven years remaining of the nine-year period, and die. We have done nothing. But the five-year survival rate looks wonderful. My point is, we have no way of knowing how much this may be affecting our very hopeful conclusions about death rate of malignancy.

"Sometimes you think that it is all a mirage, that all the things you think you've proven could be a product of your testing, of the way you take numbers."

The promising appearance, that is, could be an artifact. This particular type of statistical artifact is called lead-time bias. And there are other such statistical mirages. For example, the noted cancer biologist and writer John Cairns cited a study concerning prostate cancer in his book *Cancer: Science and Society*. The study noted that the incidence of prostate cancer in men aged seventy was about 200 per 100,000 each year, or 0.2 percent of that population. But when autopsies were done on men who had died at that age of other causes, 15 to 20 percent had microscopic, invasive prostate cancers. That means that if a new screening program had enabled discovery of these microtumors, the "cure rate" of such cancers would rise remarkably. In other words, a huge number of "new cases" of such cancer would be added to the data base, but since a large number of these would never be fatal anyway, a misleading number of new "surviving patients" would be figured into the percentages.

Cairns further notes that in terms of prediction, most people *without* cancer simply want to know what the chance is that they will die of the disease. "This is a question that we can easily answer," he writes. "From this point of view there has been no recent, major advance. The chance of dying of cancer has not altered greatly in the United States in the past 35 years."

Cairns wrote that nearly ten years ago; the statistics for the major cancers have changed little since then. The heartening cases for the cancer doctor are fewer than the depressing ones, Villar says. "Sometimes, cancer treatment is a very expensive—*very expensive*—form of psychotherapy," he says bluntly.

"But you know the one thing you cannot tell someone? You cannot tell someone, 'There is nothing more I can do for you.' That is the end, for a person, the thought that there is no hope. And that, I suppose, is the one thing a doctor cannot take from a patient—is hope. Yet that is what you would do if you said what is, sometimes, almost certainly the truth: There is nothing more I can do for you. People cannot live with that. Yet the expense is . . ." He shakes his head, presses his lips together, a man caught in a very different dilemma from the scientist's. Yet how much all these quandaries look alike after a while.

As I would see over the coming months, Villar's insight was shared by many cancer physicians who are concerned that even highly toxic treatments are ordered without evidence that they are helping, because a doctor feels, in the words of one critical medical oncologist: "I can't just let the poor lady die."

Why can't we just *see*? Why won't the picture come clear so that we can just see it, plain as day? But the world through the "macroscope" is no clearer than that through the microscope; it just has its own demonic artifacts. Try to see what cancer is doing to everyone and the picture becomes as fuzzy with error bars as when we try to see what it is doing in one person's genes.

And then the frustrating thought comes: Some day it *will* all come clear; it will all seem utterly simple, and we who could not see will seem as blind as our ancestors as they stumbled in ignorance of the infectious causes of disease, as they sickened and died of bubonic plague ignorant of the fact that filth breeds rats which carry it. Will the answer turn out to be something we could not see without greater advances in science and medicine? Or will it turn out to be one of those things that has been sitting beneath our noses, an answer that once seen, like the man in the moon, can never again *not* be seen? Who can look at the full moon and not see a human face?

3

Longhorns

From Tucson to Houston is two hard days' drive across the south-western desert, a desert teeming with its own native life, taken root in the crumbled remnants of volcanic fields: two entirely different ways of building molecule-rearranging furnaces, one growing in remnants of the other. Volcanos are easier to envision that way: cauldrons where chemicals are poured to be shaped by intense heat and pressure into new kinds of rocks of different colors and shapes, to be further shaped throughout the millennia by new pressures, winds, heat, and cold.

And the living things: a very different way of mixing chemicals, far more complex ways of matching and controlling interactions and chemical changes.

In the blast-furnace heat and pressure of the volcano, chemical molecules change shape, become different substances literally wrenched and blown into new forms. Yet energy and pressure are also what extrudes the saguaro cactus out of its native earth: the temperature of a spring day, the air pressure of a windless morning. How? Within the cells of living things, microcsopic protein molecules —enzymes—carry out chemical reactions in micromeasure, contin- uously. This allows life to exist under its strict controls in a tiny window of temperature and pressure, the climate of most of earth, where the body will not burst into flame, collapse under force. The

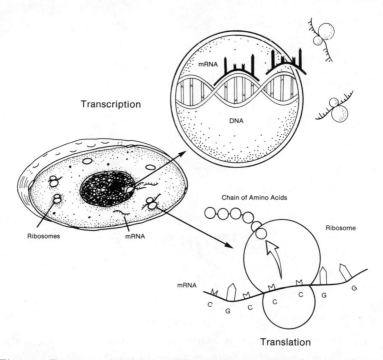

Figure 7. From gene to protein: *When a gene is activated, a complementary strand of the messenger molecule mRNA is formed against the gene in the transcription process. As depicted schematically in the upper right, during the actual transcription process, a segment of DNA splits open and a complementary mRNA molecule forms alongside it. The mRNA then slips through the nucleus into the cell cytoplasm. On the ribosomes, depicted schematically in the lower right, the RNA message is translated into the appropriate protein subunits. Called amino acids, these subunits are linked together like beads, then folded into the complex three-dimensional shapes characteristic of completed proteins.*

great director of all this activity is the DNA molecule, containing coded instructions for producing all the proteins. The construction process, in a nutshell, works like this.

When a gene segment of DNA is activated or "turns on," a related molecule is assembled alongside and up against it, matched like a key's teeth to its lock's tumblers, by the same complementarity that holds the DNA together. This newly formed molecule is called ribonucleic acid, or RNA. RNA comes in several forms; this form is called, appropriately, messenger RNA, because its job is to carry the message encoded in the DNA within the nucleus to other molecules outside the nucleus. RNA is similar to DNA in structure but is only single-stranded. The messenger-RNA molecule is the gene's transcript; the process called transcription. All this takes place within the cell's nucleus.

Now the messenger RNA slips out through the nuclear membrane. It moves to the cell's workbench, an automated factory that makes robot manufacture look primitive. Here are found structures called ribosomes, meatball-like mixtures of different kinds of RNA and proteins; these are the code readers (see Figure 7). The messenger RNA latches nose-end onto the ribosome, and as it moves along the surface of the ribosome, whichever of twenty building blocks of proteins were encoded in each segment of the messenger are pulled out of the cellular soup in precise order and linked together like a string of beads. It is on the ribosomes that the strand of messenger RNA is decoded or "translated" into a strand of protein; the process is called translation. The protein strand then folds up into any one of thousands of complex shapes, which are determined by the push and pull of its unit "beads"; these shapes in turn determine the protein's activity.

Presto: human, saguaro, fly, bacterium, virus. Presto? That much accounts for the growth and development of an organism, but not for its creation, for its shaping under the steady pressure of evolution—a process acting not during a mere gestation period but down through the millennia. Through this process an organism now and then becomes something infinitesimally different from what its heritage, as encoded in its parents' DNA, would have dictated.

Evolution operates on the same harsh rule as the forces that shape the southwestern basin and range: Mutations of living organisms, of their genetic message centers, occur randomly. Only through mutation of its DNA has any offspring ever been different than its parents' DNA dictated.

Mutations do not occur for a purpose. They are random events, accidental alterations in the makeup of the incredibly long DNA molecule. They may occur as one parent's DNA molecule is being passed on to an offspring in fertilization, as half its genetic endowment. They may occur afterward. (In one-celled organisms, any mutation would be passed on to offspring; in higher animals and

plants, only mutations in the "germ-line" or seed would be passed on.)
Occasional mutations of an organism's genes are part and parcel of
life on earth. But nearly all mutations, understandably, are fatal or at
least of no benefit to the organism or cell that inherits them. Ordinarily they represent a skewing of vital directions; at best they generally
represent a change without serious consequences for better or worse.

There is, however, a near-zero chance that a random change in
genetic message will make an organism better able to live and reproduce than its normal kindred. Near zero, but not quite zero, and
in that tiny window of probability life evolves. One time in, say, a
billion, a mutation makes dividing daughter cells able to process
food more efficiently (for example, using less energy in doing so) or
to withstand the heat of a desert noon, or the chill of night, or lack
of water. Because of that accidental benefit, such an improved mutant
survives and reproduces more daughter cells than its kindred. If it is
radically more successful, it may even outclass "normal" kindred;
they may die out while descendants of the new and better version
populate like crazy, until yet another mutation somewhere down the
long evolutionary road yields a descendant still better at living.

And that's about all the rules you need to play out the game of
evolution in your mind, those rules operating trillions of times a
second in all species around the world, down a corridor more than
two billion years long.

The whole key to evolution, a scientist once noted, lay in the
"moment" when the organism and the code for producing it were
encapsulated in the same package. That tied the success of the code
to its organism. Consider that, for it is a novel idea: The code to
generate a thing and the thing itself are bound together inside one
bubble (a cell). If the organism "works well," it spreads its code
around, which creates more of these good (by definition) organisms;
if the organism "works poorly" the code for it goes out the evolutionary window along with it.

If that seems obvious, consider that nonliving things do not work
that way. Any kind of rock represents a combination of chemicals at
a given temperature and pressure. It represents therefore a certain
code or recipe: Put iron and copper, silicon and carbon together in
such-and-such proportions at a certain temperature and pressure and

you get rock A. Rock A may last a billion years or crumble in an instant, but the recipe will neither be passed along nor lost. Meet the same conditions again and you get Rock A again, and again, and again.

The encapsulation of coding molecule (DNA) with the whole set of molecules (proteins) it encoded was a signal series of events in the development of life, perhaps the major difference between the existence of organic molecules found drifting in space and buried in ancient earth rock, and the existence of living things. But it is in turn a particular case of a much wider principle operating throughout living nature: the idea that two separate destinies may be linked for mutual benefit, the idea of cooperation. We have been aware in the century since Darwin that survival of the fittest often means that the strong devour the weak, but that is not all it entails. Biologists are more and more often citing cooperation between different organisms as a complementary idea equally essential to life.

Dr. Lewis Thomas, the eminent physician who heads the Memorial Sloan–Kettering Cancer Institute in New York City, pointed out in his book *Lives of a Cell* that in most cases of symbiosis, the joint venture benefits both host and parasite. Even when bacteria infect a host, it is more common for the bacteria to benefit or at least not harm the host than for harm to result. The bacterium *Escherichia coli* lives harmlessly in the human intestine (*coli* refers to the colon); *rhizobium* bacteria colonize the roots of some plants and make them able to fix their own nitrogen from the air so they do not need fertilizers to grow. The reason for the success of cooperation is as simple as the rules of evolution: A parasite that makes its host more successful at living will likely get itself reproduced more often, and that, after all, is *the* law of the jungle: survive and reproduce. Kill or be killed, only when it comes to that. The *rhizobium* that makes its host more adaptable and more successful provides itself more hosts. The parasite that kills its host is getting no advantage.

Early in the history of life, when the seas were full of one-celled animals, many of these cooperative ventures were undertaken (by mistake, at random, by mutation), and some worked stunningly well. Symbiotic communities grew, first colonies of several one-celled organisms, then colonies in which many cells of one type aggregated in communion with many cells of a different type. Then differences in cell type increased. The Portuguese man o'war, for example, is actually a community of distinctly different organisms living in such close symbiosis that they appear to be and are labeled as one creature.

The human body really is a colony of cooperating cells, ten trillion of them of hundreds of distinctly different types, all acting in the most precisely regulated way under the aegis of the highly successful human DNA. Each of one person's cells contains a virtually identical copy of that DNA complement, whether the cell is of the skin or liver, brain, or blood. Yet in no two people except for identical twins is the DNA complement the same.

Consider cancer in this light: One cell, of whatever type, goes out of control. The DNA message that encodes one or more of its proteins is somehow twisted; instead of growing in cooperation with other cells, this cell simply grows and divides on its own, no longer part of the colony. Some have called these "outlaw" cells, but that metaphor misses the point. There is no point. The cell isn't growing wild because it seeks something, but because it has lost something—control over its growth. Some of the most deadly cancers do not even grow rapidly; the tumors of the most fatal breast and lung cancers grow and divide extremely slowly relative to the growth and division rates of other cells, like skin and blood, and that makes them very hard to detect. They simply don't stop growing. (Slow growth also makes such cancers hard to treat with chemotherapy, because the best strategies usually involve drugs that preferentially attack dividing cells and therefore have their greatest effect on rapidly dividing tumor cells.)

To coordinate precisely the growth and operation of the ten-trillion-cell colony that is John Doe, close coordination, timing, and control are obviously of paramount importance. When Doe cuts his hand badly and bleeds a great deal, it is important for the bone marrow to produce new blood cells very rapidly until Doe has enough blood again, and then it is important that they slow down. Leukemia represents a loss of such control in production of white blood cells. The lymph system, as mentioned, is a network of fluid ducts parallel to the blood system, and lymph screens blood and cells for invading bacteria or viruses. When those foreign substances are present, certain lymph cells must grow and divide rapidly in response; then they must stop. Lymphomas, such as Hodgkin's, are the result of proliferation of certain lymph cells.

For Doe's hand to heal, it is important that skin cells grow and divide very rapidly. In the healing of a deep wound, doctors note, tissue cells proliferate so explosively that their rate of growth approximates that of some fast-growing tumors. Further, in the healing of a wound, it is important that cut blood vessels be repaired, and there are enzymes involved at such times that bring about the construction of new sections of blood vessel. When a tumor reaches a certain size, it too can activate these enzymes, and a tumor can actually call in its own blood supply to feed the growing cells deep within it. That is the reason that an unusual pulsebeat, like Villar detected in Bob Delp, can be the sign of a tumor.

A tumor, whether benign or malignant, is a colony of identical cells all descended from a single misdirected ancestor, carrying on its own life, a parasite of the John Doe colony of which it was originally a cooperating part. If it kills its host, it too will die, but again, it is not "seeking" anything; it has lost something. In fact, tumors themselves rarely kill, unless they physically interfere with the operation of other organs like the heart or lungs, or so break down an organ's tissue that it will not work any more. When cancer kills, it is usually metastatic, system-wide cancer, and then when a colonizing tumor interferes with a vital organ or a vital process like immune defense.

Biologists speak of "programmed cell death" as one of the most important features of the body. Primitive types of cells called stem cells give rise to more-differentiated cells—that is, cells that have taken up their final, specific jobs. The function of a red blood cell is to carry oxygen, of a white blood cell to attack bloodstream invaders, of a muscle cell to contract and relax. The function of a skin cell is actually to be a dead cell. In final form the skin cell is flooded with an insoluble protein, becoming a little sack of concrete to waterproof and shield the body. When you get a simple abrasion, the whole dead layer is rubbed off to expose the living, sensitive, blood-fed cells below the surface.

It is just as important that cells die on schedule as that they reproduce when needed. It is the body's way of renewing itself. Again, the cancer cell does not follow the pattern; it just keeps growing and dividing, immortal.

As would be expected, fully differentiated cells that have terminally divided cannot become cancerous (there is evidence that some cells can "de-differentiate," returning to a more primitive state, but that is not certain). Cancer is a disease of the more primitive cell types that are to divide further. An important way of staging the severity of some cancers is to determine at what stage of development its cells are. Generally, the more primitive stem cells yield the more aggressive cancers, the more differentiated cells the less aggressive, less invasive tumors.

Also as one would expect, tissues that do not continue growing in adulthood never become cancerous in adults. There are no cancers of the heart muscle itself, nor of the nerve cells of the brain, because they live out the life of the organism without further reproducing.

"Cancer cells go on potentially forever," Lew Cantley would comment one day at his Harvard lab as we talked about programmed cell death, "carrying the DNA complement of the person they were taken from for as long as you culture them. In a strange way, cancer represents immortality"—immortality at the expense of cooperation.

So, what, then, causes cancer?

Gary Gallick, a postdoctoral fellow teaching virology, is asking his graduate students that very question in the last session before 1984 spring finals. The students, in various programs at the University of Texas, have just filed into the small classroom high up in Houston's M.D. Anderson Hospital and Tumor Institute, one of the country's largest fortresses in the cancer war. In one way, Gallick says, the answer is that lots of things cause cancer, but let's try to narrow the question down and be specific.

"As a review, let's talk ourselves through the course, from the beginning," he suggests. Only three students are here at the outset: a muscular, blond young man, Mark Harvey; Alexandria Campbell, a dark-haired young woman; and Euphorbia Harrison, a slender, middle-aged black woman who is already answering Gallick's first question as the last students silently take their seats.

Gallick: "We'll be talking about oncogenes and their relationship to cancer. Virology has led us here—though not by a direct route, was it? So to start with, how do we determine that something causes a disease, that it is a disease-causing agent?" He scans the faces, jiggling a small piece of chalk.

Harrison: "First, the agent must be associated with the disease. Second, the agent must be isolated. . . ."

"Yes, exactly! And what is Ms. Harrison relating? What are these?"

Koch's postulates, she replies. Yes, there is, after all, a set of rules to be used in saying what causes or does not cause a particular disease; it is not all hit and miss by any means. Microbiologist Robert Koch postulated a set of four rules to be invoked in order to prove beyond doubt that a particular agent is the cause of a disease.

Harrison repeats: "Second, the associated agent must be isolated. Third, the agent must be inoculated into a susceptible animal, which in fact develops the disease. And finally, the agent must be recovered, or re-isolated, from the animal in which the disease is produced."

"Yes," Gallick says, "a very sound and thorough method for *proving* that agent A is the cause of disease B; not that it is merely associated with it or is a symptom, but causes it. Good, and of course we run into a major problem with using Koch's postulates in human disease, don't we? Where do we run into problems with Koch's postulates, remembering that each is vital to proving the cause? It's Number 3, isn't it? Here's the point at which we would need to reinoculate the agent into a human, show that the human in fact gets the disease, and recover the agent. We can't, we don't want to do that with humans. So we use laboratory rats, and we give them saccharine and show it gives them cancer." He adds in an aside to the visiting writer: "And everyone laughs and says that doesn't *prove* it gives humans cancer; and, of course, they're right. But I haven't heard anyone volunteering to be a guinea pig, and I don't blame them." He turns back to the class.

"Anyway, yes, we use a susceptible animal to prove that reinoculation with the suspected agent will in fact produce the disease; without that step we're merely speculating, we've merely recovered an agent associated, correlated with the disease; correlation is not cause."

Perhaps the favorite adage common to the laboratory and the clinic: Correlation is not cause. A may always appear just before B, for example, but that doesn't make A the cause of B.

Now Gallick returns to his original question, something of a theme question for this course in virology: What causes cancer? And repeats this well-known story, with some explanation:

"In the sixties, viruses were very much in vogue as causes of cancer. In the seventies they were out. Now they are returning. Viruses do cause cancer; we know that they cause cancer in animals. But why has this been so difficult to prove? Again, consider Koch's postulates," which he has written on the board.

1. Associate an agent with the disease. "The viral agent is present in very low amounts; therefore it's hard to find."

2. Isolate the agent. "Exceedingly difficult. Mouse leukemia grows ubiquitously. Human leukemia usually involves some subset of the T-cells"—types of blood cells that are a major part of the immune defense system. "A whole new technology needed to be developed to culture and challenge in an appropriate system."

The technology: genetic engineering. The appropriate system, he explains, was based on a model developed in the laboratory of Robert Weinberg with an ingenious series of experiments.

And see how the experiments follow Koch's postulates: Transform mouse cells with a carcinogen (methylcholanthrene); remove the DNA (the suspected agent); reinoculate into normal mouse cells; confirm that these become proliferative; reisolate the agent. Show that the agent will grow tumors in living mice, reisolate the DNA of these tumors, reinoculate, and so on.

Eventually, Robert Gallo of the National Cancer Institute would find human T-cell leukemia virus, HTLV, but we know that viruses do not cause most human cancers. In one sense, the problem isn't that we don't have any idea what causes cancer, Gallick points out, but that we know of too many very different things which definitely do. "What are they?"

One by one, class members rattle off known types of carcinogens.

- Environmental carcinogens, the longest known. Sir Percival Pott in 1775 determined that coal tar present in chimney soot was the culprit in the testicular cancer so common among men who had been London chimney sweeps as boys.
- Viruses, known to cause a variety of tumors in animals.
- Genetic abnormality. Clearly some cancers do run in some families, although it is equally obvious that many have no such connection.
- Radiation, a known carcinogen virtually since the discovery of x-rays. In that first generation of experimenters an extremely high incident of cancer, especially bone cancer, was noted.
- How about just plain aging? "Statistically you can show that there is a tremendous link between age and cancer," Gallick says, "and by that I don't just mean your chances increase as you get older; it's far more dramatic than that. At age eighty, in other words, in that single year you are eighty, your chances of getting some type of cancer are one hundred times greater than in the single year you were age ten. This suggests that cancer may result from an accumulation of genetic mutations over a long period." This last category would prove very important in one of the discoveries made in Weinberg's lab, one of those rare and fortunate cases in which statistical prediction and the behavior of the theoretical model would fit hand in glove.

Each of these five categories of carcinogens had been proven, and that had led to a great deal of pessimism among everyone in cancer research, for it had not been clear if the mechanisms of cancer were therefore exceedingly dissimilar. In fact, it appeared that there were even differences in the number of steps necessary for cancer. For example, on the environmental side, it has been shown that if you paint a mouse's skin with a tumor promoter like coal tar, it will not get cancer, but if you take the second step and irritate the place where the coal tar has been applied, tumors will develop—clearly a two-step process. Viruses, on the other hand, appear to cause cancer in one step.

"Now it should be clear why oncogene research has caused so

much excitement, so much optimism," Gallick continues. "Now, for the first time, when we look at this great variety of cancer-causing factors, we see that each may have the same target: the proto-oncogene. That is, the normal cellular gene which will begin behaving in the abnormal way that yields cancerous growth is the target of these various agents.

"What is novel and exciting here is that we're not talking about an infinite number of genes; in other words, we're not thinking that any 'hit' that mutates or damages any gene can lead to cancer. We may be looking at a few studyable proto-oncogenes."

And that means better possibilities of showing that the oncogenes are the causes of cancer. Koch's postulates cannot be carried out in humans, but in one sense imitating Koch's postulates is one of the goals of epidemiologists. Looking at a large group of people who already have cancer, they attempt to work backward to what common agent may have caused it. When an agent is associated, they then look forward to those cases in which the agent is known to be present to see if that agent again causes the disease. This was one method by which epidemiologists implicated smoking so solidly as a cause of cancer. They did not reinoculate people with the suspected agent; people reinoculated themselves, willingly, and the epidemiologists watched what happened to them and reported the results.

Similarly, we cannot inoculate healthy humans with oncogenes, but we can study the presence of oncogenes in human tumors and study how their activity changes as the disease develops. These efforts have proven remarkably successful in some cases, less so in others.

Gallick moves on to discuss areas of interest in his own research. He is monitoring the protein encoded by one of the known human oncogenes, called *ras*, which he has studied in various human tumors. Gallick is a postdoctoral fellow with Dr. Jordan Gutterman, a researcher with a special interest in interferon, that so-far enigmatic protein produced by the body's immune system to fight viral infections.

Gutterman, a physician, is now running clinical trials at M.D. Anderson using interferon as a weapon to reduce tumor size in critically ill patients. Because the value of interferon is still unproven, the trials involve only patients for whom all other therapy has failed, patients with no other hope.

The first person ever given interferon in a clinical trial, Chicago housewife Joan Karafotas, got her shot here in 1981 and became an instant celebrity. She was suffering from an incurable but slow-growing lymphoma, whose growth has been stopped, so far, by her interferon injections. Why not use it on everyone, then? Because it hasn't worked on everyone, although Gutterman is very excited about the wide range of tumors that have shown shrinkage during clinical trials, and he is very optimistic about the future. However, that disparity between the effects of one treatment protocol on different cancers, on the same cancers in different people, on the same cancer in the same person at different times, is one of the deep frustrations of the clinical researcher. This lack of consistency is so far without explanation.

Interferon works in a unique fashion. Most products of the body's immune system are designed to recognize foreign objects, whether viruses or bacteria, and then to take them out of action by physical means, either engulfing and devouring them or physically bonding with them so they settle out of the bloodstream. Interferon works against the genetic production line, interfering (hence the name) with the translation of some DNA into protein. Thus, although interferon action is not fully understood, it is hoped that combinations of different types of interferons eventually will combat the body's own DNA whenever an oncogene has switched on, causing uncontrolled growth.

In his office, Gutterman discusses the successes and uncertainties of the trials so far. He has found and reported many cases of remission from interferon use. One problem is that remission means that a tumor has stopped growing or, if removed, that there are no further signs of tumor development. Unfortunately, if even a few tumor cells are resistant to the drug, they will be at a great growth advantage if all the remaining tumor cells are destroyed.

That means that chemotherapy itself may *improve* the environment for any cancerous cells that can resist it, and it is one reason doctors suspect that cancers that appear destroyed by chemotherapy sometimes return, this time resistant to the drug that initially worked.

Nevertheless, Gutterman remains a firm believer that ultimately "we will manage cancer the way we manage hypertension." That is, although a single magic bullet may not be found against cancer, a variety of weapons, with interferons prominent in the arsenal, will make cancer a nonfatal, treatable disease. A single type of interferon would be less likely in a treatment protocol than just the right balance of a number of different kinds.

The drugs used to treat cancer now number in the dozens; the protocols or programs involving them and, usually, surgery and radiation treatment as well, number in the hundreds. They make up the bulk of the treatment that goes on here in a complex network of hospital buildings, classrooms, and research laboratories in several giant buildings in downtown Houston, a complex that is a small city unto itself.

The physical plant of what is called the University of Texas (UT) System Cancer Center here covers nearly two million square feet—the same floor space as in one thousand good-sized houses of two thousand square feet each. And that is not counting the ten-story clinic expansion that will add another 245,000 square feet, the eight-story research building of 132,000 square feet, the genetics lab of 4,400 square feet, or the 12,000-square-foot veterinary research laboratory being added to support the system, which already has one of the country's largest colonies of chimpanzees, used in research because the animal's immune system most closely matches humans'.

Current investment in the buildings alone is $152 million. The operating budget, separate from physical-plant cost, was $254,389,314 —more than a quarter of a billion dollars—for fiscal 1984–85.

In this citadel work 6,189 full-time employees and 731 volunteers. In 1984–85 they cared for 31,116 patients, counting both inpatients and outpatients. Every day, some 1,200 outpatients can be seen in the center's various clinics, and the several hospital buildings have 507 beds.

All for cancer. The UT System Cancer Center treats no other disease. It is only one of twenty NCI-designated "comprehensive cancer centers" around the country—some not as large; some, like Memorial Sloan–Kettering, larger. NCI also designates twenty-one other centers that are not quite as large, like the University of Arizona, as clinical cancer centers. Moreover, the centers themselves barely hint at the enormity of the American investment in cancer treatment. Only a small fraction of cancer patients are treated in centers, most of them on referral from smaller hospitals. Many, if not most, cancer patients are treated entirely by doctors in their own communities.

We treat sick people here. You might have taken the words right out of Emil Freireich's mouth. A leader in the development of chemotherapy and chairman of the M.D. Anderson hematology department, he is at the moment angry with a visiting writer who has just gotten the world backwards. In the last year, the writer had said, a lot of discoveries have been made in the laboratory that have increased our understanding of cancer.

Dr. Freireich raises a hand to interject, a gesture well known, it is said, throughout the realm of medical oncology. Freireich has a reputation as a tough combatant, a hard-nosed debater, and an outstanding chemotherapist. But after all, this is no polite, after-you-Alphonse profession, doctoring; not in any aspect of it. Doctors do not generally air their criticisms of one another in public, any more than they air disagreements over patient care in front of the patients. But they do air those disagreements, often heatedly, all the more so when they are over life-and-death issues. Sit in on a clinical conference and the air crackles with disputation.

"Stop right there," Freireich says. "First, let me tell you, discoveries are not made in the laboratory. Discoveries are made in the clinic. The clinic is the only place where discoveries can be made, where the patients are. You want to talk about basic science? Cancer treatment is the most basic of all science. And when you say chemotherapy, you are really talking all therapy. What other kind of cancer therapy is there? There is surgery, and then there is chemotherapy, whether by radiation or some other chemical activity.

"All progress in the control of disease is made in the clinic. The laboratory is a place where you codify, summarize, analyze what you have learned in the clinic. Lab research can clarify things observed in the clinic, but it cannot substitute for clinical observation.

"To learn of disease you can't just look and think. You must agitate, disturb! Leukemia wasn't discovered in a fish. Leukemia was discovered in a person! Pathology was the very beginning of experimental medicine, of research.

"Here is the beginning of medical research: A man falls down. He's dead! What killed him? Look, he has an unusual lump. You must now intervene, you must cut out the lump. It was a clinician who first saw a living patient with a lump, back in ancient times, and that clinician said, What if we cut out the lump? He did so. And the patient survived. Therapy, intervention, revealed the basic facts to be studied in the lab.

"Now look at radiation therapy. Surgeons discovered that half of those who had surgery died because they had grown new lumps. Why? Obviously, we didn't get all the cancer cells. So we'll cook those left behind. That was the beginning of radiation therapy. Radiation had great specificity in its target: You could point right at a small target and hit it. It was the beginning of chemotherapy. Radiation therapy cured cancer, cured it! Then we went to the lab, only then, and asked: Is there a differential cell kill? Does radiation kill more cancer cells than normal cells?

"Now we have chemicals with which to treat cancer. Do you know how that started? Lymphoma was treated with nitrogen mustard. Now, what in the world made someone think of using nitrogen mustard, mustard gas, a deadly poison, to kill cancer cells? That came out of World War I, from a clinical observation about the effects of nitrogen mustard on the white blood cells of its victims." Use of the chemical to treat cancer did not begin until the later stages of World War II.

"And you know what they said, the academics? 'Oh, there's no intellectual content to this at all. It's just a bunch of dumb doctors giving this stuff.'

"Fine, but let me tell you this: If we're going to make progress in the future, the smartest group must be in the clinic. The smartest guys can't be in the lab, confirming what little we already know— and we know very, very little—yet 80 percent of the research money goes to the guys who study what we already know."

To hear him, you would think Freireich was a doctor who eschewed the laboratory, who stayed clear of the complexities of science. On the contrary. His papers are as full of hard-core science as any laboratory investigator's, of the vagaries of statistical formulations, of analyses of treatment groups by various standards as a means of determining the best therapeutic protocols. This is the Freireich who,

with Emil Frei of Boston's Dana–Farber Cancer Institute, developed
the first chemotherapy protocols to succeed in combatting childhood
acute lymphocytic leukemia (ALL), one of the commonest cancers
in children and until then nearly always fatal. Their work ultimately
changed the course of the disease. More than half now are cured.

Freireich and Frei shared the prestigious Charles F. Kettering
Prize in 1983. In his acceptance speech for that prize, Freireich explained in fascinating detail how his team had analyzed groups of
patients in an attempt, eventually successful, to predict which
patients would be the most amenable to conventional therapy, who
therefore would not be good candidates for experimental protocols,
and who would most certainly fail in conventional therapy. The
speech outlines the practice of empirical science: of science taking
in-hand experience as its given, attempting to work back to the
principles that would allow one to predict—always science's ultimate
goal.

Freireich's argument isn't over whether to do science or not, but
where. The best place to look for answers is in the clinic, where the
patients are; of that Freireich has no doubt.

Is that how the scientific community views medicine? By no means,
which may account for some of Freireich's anger. This issue raised
by the visiting writer is clearly not new.

"Radiation therapists? They were considered quacks: 'All you guys
do is cook people.' Then the radiation therapists decided we were
quacks. Why? The first chemotherapy given clearly caused remission of tumors," he says, adding sarcastically, "but all the patients
died. So, clearly you couldn't cure people with chemotherapy; chemotherapy would never have the specificity of radiation therapy."

And Freireich concludes with his belief that such cure as there
will be for cancer will come from chemotherapy: "99.9 percent of
those who die of cancer have systemic cancer"—that is, cancer that
has metastasized. "Lumps don't kill people; medicine is too good for
that, we can cure lumps. Only systemic treatment will cure systemic
cancer. We can't yet discriminate between whether a tumor will or
will not metastasize, but we're learning to." And that was the general thrust of his Kettering Prize address: ALL, which he and Frei
had learned to attack successfully nearly twenty years earlier, is
systemic virtually from the outset, therefore it might serve as a proto-

type for coping with other deadly system-wide cancers—if the lessons learned were used.

"We're not going to cure cancer by giving all the money to all the molecular biologists to map out the human genome," he says, referring to a proposal that has been in the news in recent days. "But a cure is going to come. It takes clinical people to be creative, yet young people don't go into clinical research. They find it demeaning; they don't get money," he says.

"There's an excess of physicians who are really tradespeople. And on the other side the academic community just wants to study onco-genes. We have a national crisis and no one is willing to look at it and admit it. Clinical professors don't get tenure [at the University of Texas]. Academic professors get tenure, they get tenure so they can work on oncogenes."

Freireich shakes his head, his anger abated. "Do you want to accompany me on grand rounds? It should be interesting. You'll really see something."

Grand rounds is the hospital's group meeting for medical person-nel covering recent common concerns or problems to which the entire staff needs to be alerted. Today George Bodie, one of Freireich's frequent collaborators, is discussing the terrible effects of *candida* (CAN-did-a) yeast infections, and he has the slides to demonstrate that the effects of these common infectious agents on patients al-ready debilitated by cancer are indeed terrible. The slides are of pa-tients afflicted with what look like possible tumors or outbreaks of rashes associated with some tumors, followed by slides of autopsies showing the ravages of the yeast infections, which strike most often when the immune system is depressed. These infections, in other words, are often masked as cancer itself, but they can kill inde-pendently of the effects of cancer if they are not recognized and treated.

These are the front lines, plainly. Freireich watches intently, looks back at each questioner, often nods approvingly. "Good stuff," he whispers. It is only by coincidence that we are hearing this particular grand-rounds lecture, but Freireich could hardly have picked a better one to illustrate his point. *Here is what you have to look for, here is where you have to keep your eyes peeled, to be forever alert. Here, where it's a matter of life and death, you have to be right.* What is cancer? Just when you think you've got the answer, have the tests down pat, along comes something that is not cancer at all but looks just like it, to frustrate you again. Something you could discover only in the clinic.

On the road, north and eastward. The lab and the clinic, a fascinating distinction. Are they necessarily mutually exclusive? Of course not. And over the months to come the doctors and scientists I talked to would insist on as much. Pure, basic research is needed; clinical research is needed. But such acknowledgments mask a very real and basic dispute that rages now as it has for many years: Where is the answer going to come from? Where are we going to look for the answers? There is only so much money, and it is foolish not to admit that when a project over here is funded, it may be at the expense of a project over there. You pays your money and you takes your choice.

We could draft two propositions, setting the subject up for debate. We could give clear dominance, in each of two contradictory propositions, to either basic science or the applied research of the teaching hospital—and I have certainly heard enough from people on either side, enough criticism of one or the other, to know that we would not be creating an unrealistic opposition if we were to do so. Freireich is outspoken, but he says what many physicians like him will say in private and in public. He believes that both clinical and basic research need funding, but that the balance has tipped too far toward the basic.

On the other side, just weeks after my interview with Freireich, cancer researcher Lewis Cantley related an interesting anecdote then making the rounds of basic science laboratories: During the 1950s, the massive federal effort in the then-war against polio aimed at applied science, at improving iron-lung technology to aid those already suffering from the crippling disease. Had that strategy proved right, the anecdote goes, millions of people would now be sporting pocket-sized iron lungs, and we would still have no way to prevent polio.

Instead, of course, Jonas Salk, working with a few colleagues in a laboratory in competition with others across the country, around the world, found the answer; although still incurable, polio is nearly wiped out as a disease. Still incurable. Almost wholly preventable. A disturbing, provocative analogy.

In September of 1984, *Nature* magazine, the British journal that is probably the most respected of the journals that cover all branches of science, sponsored its Boston conference, "The Molecular Biology of Cancer." Perhaps in recognition of this frequent difference of viewpoint, the conference was structured so that each segment featured scientific researchers' findings followed by a physician offering the clinician's view.

Weinberg, a conference participant, commented to me beforehand: "It's a strange mixed bag . . . a rather artificial marriage. What do we have to tell one another? I can't imagine what a clinician can tell me that will help in uncovering the molecular biology of cancer, because the problems I'm interested in have to be solved at the cellular and subcellular level. This might contribute to my liberal education in biology, but I don't think it will shed much light on the problems I study."

And conversely, "I can't think what I would tell them that would change the way they now treat their patients."

Two mutually exclusive propositions, or lemmas, each of which appears independently correct, were called by the ancients a dilemma, on the horns of which could always be found the puzzled interlocutor.

Later, Freireich would make an interesting observation on this dilemma—that it should not exist, that it is an artificial one. Clinical and basic research ought to be seen as a continuum, he said, and funded as such. They are not—hence the dilemma, sui generis.

4

First Steps

Heading north through Houston, next stop the National Cancer Institute in the Washington suburb of Bethesda, Maryland, a three-day drive with a dilemma for company: What is the first step in the search for reality? Is it a burst, a serendipitous occurrence within the mind that links formerly disparate events together into an image of *how it really is,* an image that can be tested? Or is it an observation or a series of observations that lead the curious and prepared mind to turn observed events on each side, turn them inside out, sniff and poke them to see where they lead? The difference marks a frequent bone of contention between the empirical approach and, say, the model-building approach to scientific investigation.

Most molecular biologists I know are, like Weinberg, model builders, and that method of attack has its own rigors and its own dangers. How do you look for something? Build a model of what you think it is, based on what you know of it, and jam it up against the world. You have to be very honest about whether your model fits, however, and how well, and in what circumstances it has been tested. The world is full of tricks, even for the prepared mind.

But some other molecular biologists and probably most doctors are empiricists, like Freireich: The *first event* in the voyage of discovery is an event witnessed. *A man falls down. He's dead! What killed him?* Thus we begin. Or one scientist's summing up of her specialty: "Molecular genetics offers a good autopsy." Coming, as it does, after the fact.

A doctor is studying victims of war's horrors, survivors of a gas attack. He discovers that nitrogen mustard has inhibited reproduction of white blood cells; were his mind not prepared, that might mean nothing, but in his prepared mind a question arises: Might this toxin slow the reproduction of runaway white blood cells in leukemia victims? And he's off on a voyage of discovery, a voyage of rescue.

Now consider Weinberg again, back on Longfellow Bridge. Here is a man witnessing nothing but heaps of snow plowed back like frozen breakers, making him navigate with some thought a route he normally walks automatically. Boom! A model, full-formed: What if . . . ? And then the faith to doggedly pursue this creature of the mind, believing in the model's reality, poking and prodding it, forcing it to reveal itself in nature; steadfast against false appearances that confirm what you want to believe, pushing for the telling experiments that ultimately will come up binary: 1/0, right/wrong, win/ lose.

It is obvious that one approach is not right, the other wrong. Both empiricism and model-building demand diligence and hard work, disciplined study, mental alacrity, and nerve—the willingness to be wrong set against an absolute determination to be right. Nevertheless it seems to me the two represent very different ways of wrestling with the beast, of trying to find out what is real and what is not. Of course, that last is what science is all about; but it is also where science meets the rest of us, representing one way of seeking reality, and therefore one way of stating it.

Michael Wigler of Cold Spring Harbor tried to avoid virology and virologists because he found it all "somewhat pedantic." He never liked working in model systems, he told me, "especially when there's no clear connection to the larger, more interesting problem." Wigler was interested in mammalian cells, *his* real world, and wanted to learn all he could within those cells, not by studying viruses as a model system for them, as virologists do. Wigler's larger, more interesting problem was cellular biology—cytology—and to many clinicians the immediate and terrorizing case of cancer in the human body is that larger, more interesting problem.

But Wigler was quick to point out that most of the best people in molecular biology back in the 1970s were in virology. "Virology has done very well," he said, granting that most of our current knowledge of the workings of the cell have come from understanding viruses that attack cells. Why? The answer offers an interesting insight into the workings of basic science, and a clue why, to these investigators, cancer is interesting for what it tells of normal life.

* * *

Behold the virus. You cannot see it, even with the most powerful light microscope, yet its effects are visible. Investigated with the electron microscope, which approximates seeing in providing images of a kind, the structure of various viruses could indeed be beheld, tested against what the imagination made of them (see Figure 8). The virus, composed of DNA and protein, is for those reasons a living system, though whether "alive" in our understanding of the word is debatable. The virus is demonstrably *nothing more* than a DNA molecule surrounded by a protein coat. It was thus, as Wigler noted, the first life system in which it was possible to apply molecular biology. It was the perfect meeting ground between biochemistry and biology, the nexus, the point where two very different lines crossed.

DNA in its natural form is not visible under even an electron microscope. Through various staining techniques it can be seen as a long string of beads, but the beads are actually the protein with which the DNA is iced for photographing. The result is like looking at a spider web at a distance, seeing it as a string of glistening dewdrops. Looking at a virus under an electron microscope, such a strand of DNA can be seen wound and coiled inside a geometrically patterned coat, whose shape varies widely according to the type of virus represented. But that's all there is: DNA and coating molecules. Dead or alive?

To further confound the issue, viruses vary greatly in how much information they carry with them into the invaded cell. They all are parasites, needing help to reproduce and needing living cells in which to do so. Imagine viruses as interlopers at a home-construction site. New cells are being built according to the DNA blueprint of the host, cells composed of proteins and built through the mediation of enzyme proteins. The invading virus may be like a carpenter who shows up with nothing but a hammer and his own viral blueprint,

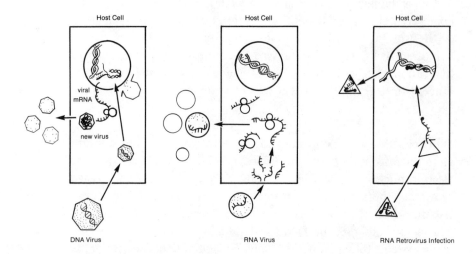

Figure 8. *Although there are thousands of different viruses, they can be broken down into three major types depending on how they get the host's genetic machinery to make new viruses. At left, DNA viruses consist of viral DNA enclosed in a protein coat. On infection, the viral DNA enters the host cell's nucleus and incorporates itself into the host's DNA. Then new virus particles are transcribed and translated along with host proteins. Center, RNA viruses consist only of RNA and a few enzymes in a protein coat. They don't need to enter the host's nucleus; they simply replicate themselves and get new viral proteins translated on the host's ribosomes to form new viruses. Most recently discovered, at right, the RNA retroviruses combine features of both other types, but they are capable of accidentally "capturing" host genes. Often mutated, these were the first instances of oncogenes discovered.*

who has to mooch everything else from the host: energy, reproductive commands, messenger RNAs. Such a virus often inserts its DNA blueprint into the host's DNA so its proteins will be translated along with the host's. But viruses also may be quite sophisticated, carrying along with them the enzymes that assemble their messenger RNAs, not needing to integrate in the host's DNA, needing only a site at which to put together new virus particles.

Some viruses do not even contain the DNA molecule, but carry their genetic message in the related RNA molecule. Some of the best-known infectious agents are such RNA viruses, including those for the common cold, rabies, and polio. But a small subset of these RNA viruses go through curious acrobatics in getting themselves reproduced. They carry into invaded cells an enzyme called reverse transcriptase, which does just what the name states, transcribing the appropriate DNA molecule out of the viral RNA, the copy-DNA then transcribed by the host in normal fashion to yield virus proteins. This latter class of RNA viruses is called retroviruses. David Baltimore shared the 1975 Nobel Prize for finding this vital key to re-creating genes out of their RNA messengers. However, the discovery produced much more than that; tumors produced by retroviruses turned out to hold the secrets to the early chapters of the oncogene story.

Imagine yourself back in the Astrodome-sized cell, the nucleus a giant sphere the diameter of the entire infield, when a virus intrudes. It will be anywhere from the size of a butterfly to a light aircraft. Most animal viruses are small compared to the cell size and carry their protein coats into the cell. Bacterial viruses generally do not; they hunker up against the cell surface and squirt their DNA into the cell's interior.

What follows is a primitive form of genetic engineering, and the understanding of the process helped create that field. Whether by sophisticated or simple means, depending on the virus, the host cell helps reproduce viral DNA and a new protein coat. New viruses created through subversion of the host's reproductive machinery spread throughout the host organism. And some of these viruses cause cancer.

*   *   *

In the late 1960s, some surprising genetic coincidences began to emerge in viruses, discovered by George Todaro and R. J. Huebner. They located gene sequences in mice that had embedded within them the instructions for making certain RNA tumor viruses. This was a major turning point in the search for cancer viruses: Genes associated with them now had been located in the *hereditary* DNA of a mammal known to become infected with this virus.

Unfortunately, as Weinberg relates that period, the wrong conclusions were drawn from the discovery. Latent, cancer-causing gene sequences had indeed been found. But many of those following the experiments assumed, as Huebner and Todaro did, that activation of this latent tumor virus caused cancer in the infected animals; this continued and intensified the belief that the virus was the cause of the cancer. Thinking in this period, Weinberg says, "was totally confused . . . by virtue of the fact details of the Huebner–Todaro model were taken too seriously."

It remained for Michael Bishop and his partner Harold Varmus at the University of California–San Francisco to begin piecing the details together in the right order. In fact, the truth, as it appears now, is considerably more fantastic than the model posed by Huebner and Todaro.

The RNA viral oncogenes did not originate in viruses. They represent, consistently, gene sequences of host organisms which at some point in evolutionary history have been *captured* from the hosts by the viruses, and have persisted. This model emerged: Purely by accident—as all mutations occur in nature—at some moment when a host cell was dutifully reading out the viral genes to produce a new virus, one of the host's own genes was accidentally read into the script. That meant that this new batch of viruses now contained the few genes instructing in the manufacture of a new virus-plus-protein-coat, *and* an extra gene of the host (see Figure 9).

The question is, why was this capture successful? That is, what did the host–gene insertion provide the virus that enabled it to compete and survive among its nonmutated brethren? Not much.

The captured oncogenes turned out to be almost perfect copies of genes that controlled the *host's* growth and division. And they did not persist very well. Viruses are so small, so economically packed, that there is no space for inserted genes that do not directly relate to their existence. These RNA viruses were crippled; the genes coding for their own reproduction turned out to be broken up by insertion of the host cell's gene. These viruses existed only in the presence of helper viruses, which could control reproduction. But they caused tumors in virtually any host they infected.

Such RNA tumor viruses thus turned out to be unsuccessful viruses, for the most part, but they were vital messengers: They carried tumor-causing genes that had been randomly captured from their hosts. In rapid succession many more oncogenes were located in these tumor viruses, each, it is now believed, representing either a host's cancer-causing gene or a normal host gene that has been mu-

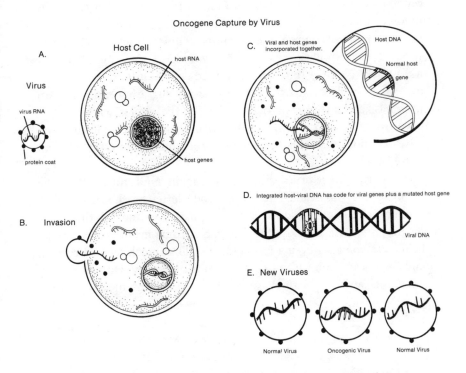

Oncogene Capture by Virus

Figure 9. How oncogene action might occur. Not every step in the process is clear, but it is known that the retroviral RNA carries reverse transcriptase, an enzyme that makes a copy-DNA to integrate into the host's genes. Sometimes this DNA apparently is read into the host in such a way that a usually-normal host gene somehow becomes incorporated into the middle of the viral DNA and later mutated, then is read out into the new virus particle as an oncogene.

tated to cause cancer. Sounding like the names of ancient deities, these oncogenes bear acronymic names recalling the organisms in which they were found. There is *src*, the one Bishop and Varmus found, standing for "sarcoma"; *ras*, perhaps the best known and most powerful, from rat sarcoma virus, and *mos*, of Moloney sarcoma virus; *myc* and *myb*; *erbB* of avian erythroblastoma, *B-lym* of lymphoma, and a whole range of transforming sequences from a variety of other animals' viruses and tumors. More than twenty oncogenes have now been discovered, virtually all first spotted within the genomes of the RNA tumor viruses, where they had accidentally become embedded.

Every new viral oncogene with its cellular counterpart offered stronger and stronger evidence that virologists were on track; but what track? None of those viruses caused cancer in humans. Virology more than ever seemed to many to be moving away from the real world. Like elementary-particle physicists, the virologists seemed to have come up with a world of minutiae of interest chiefly to themselves. Various scientists became expert in the structures of different oncogenes.

In the laboratory of Edward Scolnick at the NCI, for example, the *ras* oncogene was studied to its last code letter by the early 1980s. Scolnick and his colleagues created a map that showed the entire *ras* makeup, base by base. But had rat sarcoma ever given a human being a sarcoma, or even a bad cold? No. That much seemed certain, and there was not a whit of evidence to the contrary. Human cancers were not caused by viruses, so what was the point of all this viral study?

5

The Campus

The National Cancer Institute is a large and well-funded arm of the National Institutes of Health, which is located on a pleasant rolling campus in suburban Bethesda, Maryland, a forty-minute subway ride from downtown Washington. It is an interesting place. First, it is the funnel for nearly all the federal funds involved in cancer research and treatment that flow outward to hospitals, universities, and other research laboratories across the country, for educational programs, for anything related to cancer. Just as important, it is a research and treatment center of major proportions in its own right; many of the seminal experiments, in both basic and clinical science related to cancer, are done here. It was here that Edward Scolnick enumerated the map of *ras*, here that Robert Gallo found human T-cell leukemia virus I and later HTLV III, the cause of acquired immune deficiency syndrome (AIDS), and work in other laboratories here will be seen to be of major importance to later chapters in the search for the causes of cancer.

George Khoury, chief of molecular virology, came to the NCI in 1971 after finishing his internship as a medical doctor at Massachusetts General Hospital. He'd planned to remain two years, then return to Massachusetts Eye and Ear Infirmary to complete a residency in ophthalmology. He never made it. Khoury got hooked on the heady research atmosphere of the NCI, then on the verge of its best days, just as the war on cancer was proclaimed in 1971 by then-President Richard Nixon, and the NCI was split off as a major institute with its own congressionally authorized budget.

The basic research drew Khoury and many others, and he points out that the "system" he was studying promised basic knowledge about gene controls. That system was SV40—simian virus number 40, by someone's count. Every major molecular biologist today can trace part of his or her intellectual development to the study of this virus, which does not even cause cancer in normal cells but will induce transformation in some cell lines. Khoury refers to it the way most scientists do: "I started in SV40"—as though it were a place. In some ways it is: a place in mind space, a whole set of complex, abstract intellectual truths discovered in the study of a virus invisible in all but the electron microscope.

SV 40: "It was of interest to cancer, sure," Khoury says. "But it was the regulation of genes that the basic research with SV40 offered." With that basic knowledge came more knowledge of the loss of control involved in cancer. Neither Khoury nor others expected a sudden find of a human cancer virus, nor was one forthcoming.

In those days, it is often heard around here, the National Institutes of Health was drawing many of the best and the brightest of M.D.s into research because by serving here one became an officer in the Public Health Service, an alternative to the doctor draft of the Vietnam war, a war a great many of those who came opposed.

Asked to name the "alumni" of that period, Khoury rattles off a who's who of current cancer research: George Todaro, now scientific director of the Oncogene Co. of Seattle; Stuart Aaronson, now chief of the NCI's laboratory of cellular and molecular biology; Philip Leder of Harvard; Edward Scolnick, here until recently and now vice president of Merck, Sharp and Dohme and the company's frequent spokesman; Michael Bishop, and Harold Varmus.

"The list goes on and on," Khoury says. "The thing that's unfortunate is that a lot of young doctors now, who might have been exposed to this kind of exciting research, never get to see it."

They came to study cancer, but the secret of cancer was an ultimate goal. More immediately, in the days before the first gene had been cloned, before recombinant DNA was a reality, they came to study the viruses that many were certain were the root cause of all cancer.

Although that ultimately proved wrong, the central belief of Khoury and many others proved right—knowledge of viruses is the root of knowledge of cancer.

Khoury took me on a short tour of the rooms adjoining his lab, rooms that are now an oddity of history, a monument to a detour, however brief: windowless labs with rubber-sealed doors and showers on both sides. "These were originally planned to be 'clean' rooms," he says. "The idea then was that we would have to conduct cancer research under the most rigid containment conditions, to prevent the human cancer viruses from escaping. You would have to shower [going] in, shower [going] out."

On his wall, behind his head now as he leans back at his desk, is a poster from a symposium held in Pittsburgh a few months earlier, and there is an important personal story for him and Weinberg connected with that poster. For the present, suffice it to say that Khoury and Weinberg, both now in their early forties, grew up together in the same neighborhood in Pittsburgh in the 1950s. That two of the country's most respected cancer researchers should have known each other as children is quite a coincidence. This poster involves more than a coincidence, but the telling of it came later, as Weinberg and I talked in late summer 1984; the retelling has to come later, too, involving as it does the mysterious origins of knowledge, coincidence, serendipity, whatever makes things click.

I haven't come far enough yet to dwell on coincidence, and it's not nearly time to speak of serendipity, the wonderful and mysterious notion that hovers over the scientific laboratory like a household deity.

The basic researchers, M.D. or Ph.D., who flocked to the NCI in the early 1970s each came to take part in the drive to understand the basic mechanisms of gene regulation. The structure of DNA itself, remember, had only been elucidated in 1953. It took most of the 1960s for molecular biologists to understand the rough details of how the message encoded on the genes was ultimately translated into proteins, whether cell-building proteins or the enzymatic proteins that regulate the cell's chemistry. In the middle 1960s, the genetic code was cracked, a code no more difficult to read than any numerical table. The genetic code is a translating code from the language of DNA base units to the language of protein building blocks, nothing more. Using it, a scientist could now analyze DNA for its sequence of bases and immediately translate that into the sequence of protein building blocks that the DNA sequence called for.

But it was becoming increasingly apparent that molecular biology was only beginning to understand the complexities of the "magic molecule" DNA. For example, nearly all the 100,000 genes in the human DNA blueprint were "silent" nearly all the time. That is, they were not being "expressed" to yield proteins in these silent periods. Further, some proteins were obviously needed in great quantity and others in minuscule amounts. Then there was the fact that some proteins were not needed at all at one time, then might suddenly be needed in huge amounts.

Thus, the major terra incognita, vast and barely explored, its limits not even understood, was gene regulation. How were the genes regulated so that the gene coding for the immune system's immunoglobulin would be switched on and off frequently, as needed, while the genes coding for the growth and division of nerve cells of the brain would shut down at a certain point in development and never turn on again?

It was on the very edge of this great, exciting new territory that the young scientists found themselves. And the first thing you want to create when you find yourself in a new land is a map. To molecular biologists, a virus like SV40 is a model, a system: an analog of the models we've been building in the mind-theater, though an analog far more complex. But you can think of that model as a schematic diagram of more complex systems. In other words, the investigators into SV40—and a whole range of other equally obscure-sounding viruses—hoped that they had a microcosmic map of the larger world, understanding which they could proceed with confidence. They found in these viruses models, for example, of the ways genes regulate cell behavior, systems for studying the ways in which some cells are transformed by some genetic elements.

They studied viruses because they all contained relatively few genes, and therefore their regulatory mechanisms were neither terribly complicated nor buried in complex surroundings.

SV40 is a DNA tumor virus, a simpler model than the RNA viruses for studying gene regulation. Khoury pointed out that those studying the RNA tumor viruses—retroviruses—were involved with what then seemed more obscure systems, because it was unknown what connection they could have to cellular genes. The known RNA viruses acted in the cellular cytoplasm; having no DNA they couldn't get into the nucleus to integrate with the host's DNA. When David Baltimore discovered reverse transcriptase in 1970, suddenly a whole class of RNA viruses could be found which could *make* DNA once inside the cell—the retroviruses.

Still, retroviruses were quite obscure in the early 1970s, and many people believed they would remain an oddity, something that when fathomed might provide a small piece of the vast problem of growth and development but no more than that. In the end, they would prove to be the system most fruitful in uncovering clues to the cancer pathway. But—and this is an important, recurring pattern in science, an element in "serendipity"—many of the tools and techniques discovered through study of the DNA viruses would in turn make it possible to learn the nature of the RNA tumor viruses.

SV40 had many virtues. It contained only a few genes, and these genes were "turned on" at discrete, observable times during the viral infection. The virus was easy to propagate and relatively easy to work with and it offered the possibility of a good deal of knowledge of basic gene controls. For some of those reasons, SV40 was the system proposed for the first recombinant DNA experiment in 1973, by Paul Berg of Stanford. Berg later won the Nobel Prize for his landmark work in the development of genetic engineering—mixing, or recombining, pieces of DNA from different hosts to form genetically altered organisms. His proposal led to heated debate in the scientific community over whether such genetic engineering should be allowed, for there was a great deal of concern among scientists that a hybrid virus or bacterium might gain powers unknown in their natural varieties and might unleash new plagues on mankind. While that debate went on, for a period of about three years, gene-cloning experiments were severely restricted, and precisely the type that Weinberg needed to do were not permitted at all.

That delayed until about 1976 the viral work that formed the background for the experiments with which this story is concerned, the experiments of the later 1970s and 1980s by Bishop and Varmus, then Weinberg, Wigler, and several investigators at the NCI and at Harvard. By the winter of 1978, when Weinberg's brainstorm came,

it was possible only to speak of "transforming principles" within organisms; the term *oncogene*, put into use by Bishop, was still a much-
disputed intellectual concept with no discernible universal application in cancer. If many virologists were arguing that viruses caused
cancer, others argued with equal force that the causes of cancer were
environmental, of chemical origin, and further that they were "epigenetic": They did their work outside the genetic, DNA system.

Then came the falling-out of the late 1970s, when the virologists'
claims of the usefulness of their models fell on doubting ears. That
resulted in a large-scale exodus from the NCI, according to many
here at that time, of many of those who had come to study virology
as the war against cancer wound into gear.

And that puts into an interesting context the remarkable series
of experiments that began with the transformation of mouse cells
performed in Weinberg's lab. By the late 1970s, as noted earlier,
virologists were routinely using viruses to induce tumors in mice,
then using those virus-laden tumor cells to infect other cells in serial
progression. Furthermore, by then Bruce Ames had linked the ability
of chemicals to make cells cancerous to their ability to cause genetic
mutation in bacteria, and that was certainly an important connection, important evidence that whether chemical or viral in origin, the
action of these carcinogens was directed against genetic targets.

But it remained for Weinberg the virologist to use cellular DNA,
not viruses, to transfect cells, then to show that you could keep
reisolating the transforming principle within that naked DNA, without either virus or chemical present.

That was the beginning, as auspicious and as controversial as any
major beginning. But all that was proven in those initial cell transfections was that "something genetic" was able to cause transformation in the NIH3t3 mouse cells, the cell line created from NCI-bred
mice. Other laboratories were close behind Weinberg's, naturally,
and over the next years their names would figure in virtually every
discovery concerning the genetic nature of cancer: Wigler at Cold
Spring Harbor, Geoffrey Cooper of the Dana–Farber Cancer Institute
and Harvard, and Mariano Barbacid of the NCI. Naturally there
would be a host of other names that would figure in one or more
experiments, but those four labs were involved in nearly all of them.

There were certain questions that suggested themselves in those initial transformations. Perhaps it was only mouse cells of that particular type that would cause transformation of other such mouse cells. No; over the next few years, Weinberg's Wigler's, and Cooper's lab found that a whole series of *human* tumors' DNA also could be serially transfected into mouse cells and would cause transformation. This was significant because it showed that whatever these oncogenes looked like in terms of their base sequence, they were capable of doing what few other genetic elements would: operate in a variety of tissues and across the boundaries of species. Cells from human bladder carcinomas, lung cancer, and various human sarcomas all would transform mouse cells, and their transforming genes would continue transforming new cell cultures.

Next question: How could these oncogene sequences be isolated so that they could be identified and studied in detail? Therein lay an intimidating challenge. The mammalian genome, or DNA complement, contains about 100,000 genes, and the only thing known of the small number of oncogenes was that they transformed cells; nothing of their base sequences or functions was known. Weinberg, Wigler, and Barbacid all found the answer, each using a different method. Weinberg noted that the fact that three different laboratories found the oncogene by three different methods was, in effect, a triangulation to further establish the credibility of the concept of the oncogene model of cellular cancerous transformation.

Weinberg has always been particularly pleased with the method Chiaho Shih used in his own lab. Shih constructed a probe that they hoped would enter the jungle of mouse DNA and identify the oncogenic, transforming bits by recognizing them as human. The "bait" for the probe was made of genes from a human tumor; for all the similarity among all mammalian DNA, human DNA has a base sequence called *alu*, which mouse DNA does not. Even better, the *alu* sequence occurs very frequently, about once every six thousand base pairs. That means that nearly every human gene-sized fragment would have an *alu* sequence. Shih's probe used the *alu* sequence like a magnet, to find its partner in the human oncogene embedded in the mouse DNA.

That would be of engineering interest only, but it would turn out much later to show the fascinating way that scientific methods repeat themselves, how a method that works gets used over and over— sometimes too often, but in this case, just right—to isolate a gene that had caused a metastasis.

The strategy worked; Shih succeeded. At about the same time, investigators in Barbacid's and Wigler's labs isolated the same onco- gene. They had trapped it, yet still had no idea what it was they had isolated, that is, how the base-pair code of this oncogene would read. At this point, these scientists were convinced that they had found in oncogenes the native genes of animals that would lead to cancer, at least in the laboratory, and that included the ability to induce tumors in laboratory mice—and that is still an important distinction. They also knew that these genes were not normal. They didn't cause cancer until mutated with a chemical, and otherwise they could only be found in tumor cells. What was the relationship of these onco- genes to their normal cellular counterparts? That is, by what change in the cellular proto-oncogene could you arrive at an oncogene? And equally important, what is the biological function of the normal cellular gene that gives rise to the oncogene?

Over the years, molecular biologists have developed many different techniques for probing DNA's genetic information, all based on the physical nature of the molecule. A few weeks after I left the NCI, Lew Cantley said, in defining the basic strategy of the molecular biologist, "The trick is to make biology do the work for you; put biology's way of doing things to work and don't try to force it your way." Nature has worked out these ways of doing things over a few billion years. Play nature's game. The experiments carried out by investigators in Weinberg's laboratory are perfect illustrations of that strategy.

DNA is a double coil, zipped together by its bases into a spiral staircase. Without much difficulty, scientists can make the molecule unzip, yielding two single strands, each the complement of the other.

Let's take a simple example, remembering that DNA and the genes composing it are made of sequences of the four bases A, G, C, and T, and that the particular order of bases identifies the gene just as a sequence of letters identifies a word in English. We might wind up with a tiny bit on strand 1 that reads: AAGTC. The corre- sponding segment on strand 2, which had been opposite in the double helix, then would have to read TTCAG, following the rule that A always binds to T and G to C. Although the practice is more complex than this, you can see that if you're trying to find out if two DNA gene sequences are complementary, you can take a strand from one sequence, the complementary strand from another sequence, and put them together in solution. If they zip back up into a double helix, they're "homologous," they are very nearly the same gene; if they do not rejoin, they're not the same.

So: In the test tube in my left hand I hold one strand of the known human-bladder cancer oncogene; in my right, the entire 100,000 genes of any human cell, similarly unzipped into separate strands. Now I tag the known cancer gene in my left hand with a radioactive probe—in effect, I tack a light on it. I mix the contents of the two tubes together, and now analyze the results on photographic plates. Where the radioactive probe has burned a bright spot on the plate, I know the oncogene has annealed, or joined, to that long human DNA strand. I don't know the name of the gene it has stuck to or its function, but that isn't important, yet. It's there, it's found its home in the human genome.

(This ability of two similar genes to hybridize is used in so-called Southern blot experiments that will be seen to be vitally important technology to cancer-gene research.)

Next question: How much like the normal gene is the oncogene that has annealed to it? In other words, what mutation occurs in a normal gene to make it oncogenic? Graduate student Clifford Tabin and co-workers in Weinberg's lab spliced end to end bits of normal gene and bits of the oncogene. The combination still transformed. Gradually, they replaced more and more of the oncogene in "mix and match" experiments, trying to see how far they could go in replacing oncogenic sequences before the hybrid would not transform—that is, they wanted to isolate the smallest sequence of the oncogene responsible for transformation; that would tell them the difference between normal and cancer genes. Eventually, out of millions of base pairs, they got down to a DNA sequence just 350 base pairs long, which, as part of an otherwise normal gene, would cause transformation. Somewhere in those 350 base pairs, there had to be a difference from the norm.

That difference turned out to be incredible: Ravi Dhar at the NCI discovered that between the normal gene and the mutated oncogene there was *one different base*: the normal gene's G (guanine) becomes a T (thymine) in the cancer-producing gene. In other words, it takes a mutation of only one letter in the entire genetic message of that gene to make it an oncogene. In fact, the substitution–mutation was found in the gene sequence I used as an example earlier:

C–C–G–C–A–G–C–C–A normal gene

became

C–C–T–C–A–G–C–C–A oncogene

It was still thought—correctly, as it turned out—that it might take the action of many oncogenes to cause transformation, but here was the difference in one of them, and it was painfully small.

This was not the first time it had been shown that a small change in genes could lead to a major effect in an organism. It has long been known, for example, that a single such "point mutation" in the gene coding for the hemoglobin protein of the blood causes the often fatal condition known as sickle cell anemia, and such point mutations also cause other genetic diseases. Here was a case in which a point mutation had been implicated in cancer—not a cancer of chickens or mice, but a cancer of humans.

The next task was one of the most difficult. The sequence of the cancer gene had to be determined. It had been shown that a guanine in the proto-oncogene became a thymine in the oncogene. But genes, as noted, can be anywhere from 1,000 to 40,000 such "letters" long. Weinberg, along with other labs hot on the oncogene trail, set out on the long, arduous task of finding the sequence of the human bladder cancer oncogene. It was a search many thought might take years; it ended within months.

The answer was not the one Weinberg had wanted or expected. As one colleague pointed out, "We all felt this was a whole new kind of gene, and of course that was what Bob hoped and believed he had found, like an astronomer finding a new planet." The answer was not the one Wigler wanted, either. He had been trying to avoid the virologists for all these years, and despite close encounters thought he might be safe.

To begin with, Luis Parada, a new graduate student in Weinberg's lab in 1979, drew the kind of assignment new graduate students often do. He was to conduct a series of experiments that were important but routine, long, and—given what was expected at the other end—not very exciting. The exciting work was being done by others in the lab who were trying to sequence the human oncogene, to trap and name the beast. Parada's job was to perform what he refers to as the negative-control experiments: to compare the human oncogene with each of the more than twenty known viral oncogenes, in turn. The method was the by-then conceptually simple one of hybridizing two separated strands of DNA to see how strongly they would zip themselves back together, via Southern blot experiments.

Parada would take one strand of the unzipped human bladder oncogene in one test tube and one strand of any of the twenty known viral oncogenes in the other, and mix them together. Then he would check the results to see if they had reannealed, zipped up.

The blot technique, invented in Scotland by E. M. Southern, is fascinating in its homespun simplicity, as will be seen later; the lessons learned are of profound importance and can be learned in no other way. For now suffice it to say that these were time-consuming experiments, and Parada slogged on with neither results nor expectations of any. Everyone was sure that there was no resemblance between the human-bladder cancer oncogene and any viral oncogene.

Weinberg says a bit ruefully, "We might have had the answer sooner were it not for my skepticism. I didn't believe we would find a homology, and I think my skepticism influenced the graduate student."

The answer came with a shock: Parada found a solid match between the oncogene from a human bladder cancer and the *ras* viral oncogene, that obscure cause of sarcomas in rats. Although unexpected, in the long run this answer was far more significant than the opposite finding would have been. In fact, it changed everything.

Edward Scolnick and his associates at the NCI were the world experts on *ras*. They knew its structure to the last base and its behavior under virtually all conditions. No one had known any of the base pairs of the human oncogene—or so they had thought. Until the match.

"It was as though you had something in a black box that you

couldn't figure out for the life of you," Weinberg remembers, "and suddenly you found out it was identical to something you knew perfectly."

Mitchell Goldfarb, who had worked with the *ras* viral oncogene in Weinberg's lab, was now in Wigler's laboratory as a postdoctoral fellow, working on the "mysterious" human bladder oncogene. Suddenly Weinberg telephoned and announced to Goldfarb: "Guess what? You've been working on the same gene there as you were here." Weinberg recalls that although his lab announced the discovery first it was Cooper who was first to publish.

Wigler observes of Weinberg's find, "He was hoping to break new ground, which he was, but not as new ground as he thought, because he was in fact digging in his own backyard. A lot of irony in that."

And a lot of irony in Wigler's own disappointment when *ras* and the human tumor gene were revealed as one: "On the one hand it was good because there was already something known about those viral genes, so it was good for the field. But it was disappointing personally, because it meant that I would have to be competing with a group of scientists that I didn't particularly want to compete with" —the virologists again.

If Weinberg was disappointed, it was not for long. It took no time for him to realize the implications of this singularity and what it would mean in particular to researchers like Scolnick, patiently studying an arcane oncogene year after year, gleaning knowledge many thought would have no particular practical value.

Weinberg put a bottle of champagne in a Styrofoam container, hopped the shuttle flight to the NCI, and had Scolnick call his team together. Then he pulled out the champagne and offered a toast to those who had discovered the sequence of the first human cancer gene—in its viral manifestation.

That homology alone justified ten years and millions of dollars of funding of viral research. Every lesson learned from the oncogene in that viral model was now a lesson of human cancer—at least, it was a lesson of a human oncogene that now would be called *ras*; the role of oncogenes in human cancer was still in debate.

Had any human ever caught cancer from rat sarcoma virus? Not exactly. But the same twisted gene which, captured by that virus, caused cancer in rats had now been implicated in a human cancer.

There was at last a single common thread. Though far from a conclusion, it was a good place to begin.

This was about the time that Hartmut Land arrived in Weinberg's MIT lab, doctorate in hand, to begin his postdoctoral research. Fresh from the Max Planck Institute in Berlin, he remembers discovering, as everyone who has studied a language in school does, that his English was not as good as he had thought, especially in the mix of dialects and accents found in most American cities, and in university towns in particular. He hit it off with his benchmate, Luis Parada, himself from Colombia, South America. That would prove a useful collaboration, leading to the next in the chain of experiments that Weinberg considers the most important in his lab, that would answer the question that had lingered over the years since the first transformations: Why wouldn't *ras* transform ordinary cells? Why would it consistently transform NIH3t3 mouse cells but never normal cells of the same type? You might put the answer this way: Like Land, *ras* needed cooperation, and like Land found it close by.

PART II

REAL
WORLDS

6

Critical Mass

If sprawling Houston is the New West with its bigness, too-rapid growth, and the glitter of the Astrodome and NASA's Mission Control, Boston and Cambridge are the Old East. Colonial brick and granite, fluted columns, wooden gingerbread of the Victorian era on the back streets, the two cities separated by the Charles River and linked by a series of old stone bridges. And here are many of the first halls of ivy, starting with the first university in America, Harvard, nested in a tight warren of streets and alleys, the focus of several radial streets, an impossible network of one-way streets and a square jammed with vehicles and pedestrians challenging each other's access day and night. Across the river in Boston is the Harvard Business School, and then a little farther southeast, along broad Commonwealth Avenue split down the middle by the trolley tracks, giant Boston University. Tightly packed within this metropolitan area there are probably more colleges and universities, medical colleges, and teaching hospitals than anywhere else in the world—according to an estimate, more than sixty separate four-year institutions of higher learning. The common wisdom is that when the spring term ends in June (always late in the East, early in the West) about 100,000 people leave town; and in September, when classes start, 100,000 move in.

None of this is off the point. There is a critical mass of academic brainpower here that could find its match nowhere else, and the sheer quantity of talent is a major draw for more talent. In biology and medicine, consider this array: Sprawling in the middle of Harvard, a few blocks off Harvard Square, is the Harvard Biological Laboratories building, its front made imposing by two life-sized bronze rhinoceroses. Here much of the classic early work in genetic engineering was done, and major research is going on now in all areas of molecular biology. Massachusetts Avenue, Cambridge's main street, makes an oblique turn at Harvard, first paralleling the Charles River, then bisecting the winding river at the Harvard Bridge at the edge of the MIT campus; before crossing the bridge you can glimpse the long, massive stone building with its giant-columned portico and green dome that is MIT's trademark. Several blocks to the east, on a side street in an unimposing building that once was a chocolate factory, is the MIT Center for Cancer Research, where Robert Weinberg, David Baltimore, and many others have their laboratories.

Across the river in Boston is the Massachusetts General Hospital, a large teaching and research hospital, and south through Boston a few miles, past Fenway Park, is the intense concentration of medical facilities known as the Longwood Medical Area, including six major hospitals ranging from the Dana–Farber Cancer Institute to the Joslin Diabetes Center, as well as Harvard Medical School. Tufts Medical School is also in Boston, although the university itself is out in suburban Medford.

For Hartmut Land, all this was of considerable import when he was considering his options for postdoctoral research, although by that time the laboratory of Robert Weinberg was sufficiently well known that it was its own draw. To attract the best young scientists to an area, offerings in the arts and music and the nearness of other top scientists are always important. Land and Luis Parada are now entering their last year here, although Parada is only completing doctoral work and already knows that in a year he will go to Paris as a postdoctoral fellow. "Huki," as Land is universally known, already had his doctorate when he arrived here at the MIT cancer center. That was in March 1982. Parada and one other student have been here the longest; he arrived in November 1979 after beginning his doctoral studies that fall.

Parada and Land are as unlike in appearance and background as two men could be, yet that in itself is typical of laboratories in molecular biology. Parada, always in cutoff jeans and T-shirt, reached this high place in his career, by his own account, through a series of right choices and incredible good fortune. Serendipity, he says. Serendipity means stumbling across something of value by sheer luck, but the element of serendipity that separates it from pure dumb luck and makes it a favorite term in science is this: You were looking for something—looking hard, using all your ability, to find something important. You get more good fortune than you bargained for, but you were working hard to begin with, not idling.

Consider Parada. He comes from a middle-class Colombian family whose father pulled himself out of poverty to become an officer in the army. Parada became the first person in his family to get a college degree, but that in itself was a long way down the road from home. (His father technically beat him, returning to school after military retirement.) Parada entered the United States to study acting, going first to Milwaukee and the University of Wisconsin. To support himself, he got a job working as a technician in a laboratory at a Sears Die-Hard Battery factory. As time went on, he was drawn to science. He liked the investigative nature of the laboratory, and when he took his first biology course, already a junior in college, he decided that was the science he wanted to do. He was already twenty-four years old in 1976 when he first learned what a gene was. Luckily, he was at one of the country's best universities for biological studies. He switched over to the renowned Madison campus and won a scholarship so he could study full time. Completing his degree, he decided to apply to graduate school at MIT.

"For me, MIT was just the best, the finest school in the world," he says, leaning back against the stone-topped laboratory bench he shares with Land. "I decided if I could get in here, I'd get a doctorate; if not, the hell with it." Arriving in Weinberg's lab, he drew what appeared to be little more than a long and routine series of experiments, matching up viral oncogenes with genes from human bladder cancer, hoping to find what Weinberg himself was skeptical of.

Parada and other veterans of the lab draw a distinction between the old-timers and the newcomers. Now Weinberg is famous; the competition to get into his laboratory is stiff. At the time Parada came, another veteran recalls, it was not so difficult to get into Weinberg's lab as a graduate student or postdoc—you just had to be picked by Weinberg, and although he had his own tough criteria, there was competition only against Weinberg's standards. But Parada says that by and large the older group was more innovative, hungrier, more anxious to break new ground. He says this in complimenting Land: "He's been the most innovative of the new people." Serendipity: While a doctoral student at the Max Planck Institute in Berlin, Land had met Paula Traktman at a conference in West Germany. He said he was looking for a place to do his postdoc. Traktman convinced him that he could do no better than to apply to Weinberg's lab, and he did so.

Land is a towering Hessian. "He's as strong as he looks," a friend says, and he looks very strong. With his flowing beard and mane, dressed in the green bib overalls that are his daily attire, he looks like a German farmer or carpenter, soft-spoken and good-humored. Today he is both farmer and carpenter, though the world in which he is building and farming is one that none of us will ever see, but whose effects shape so much of our lives. Land is trying to build a pair of working oncogenes. In 1984, more than a year after he built the first, this is still no mean feat.

Land came to Weinberg's lab to work in rat embryo fibroblasts, a mouthful of a title for an important type of experimental system. Fibroblasts are connective-tissue cells, part of the network of support that molds jelly-bag cells into tissues of given shape, texture, and strength. NIH3t3 cells are fibroblasts, but they have been immortalized, made able to divide continuously without limit for experimental purposes, and no one is quite sure what other effects on cell behavior have been wrought in that change. Land's aim was to test the action of oncogenes in normal cells, in this case fibroblasts, and that presented a whole series of new problems.

Consider this experimental contrast. Unlike animal cells, bacteria are easy to grow; one-celled organisms, they need only sugar-water and nutrient to multiply like crazy. For that reason, for much basic research they are the favored laboratory systems. Some *E. coli* bacteria, for example, divide once every twenty minutes. At that rate, one cell will give rise to billions in just twelve hours, and if you conduct a genetic-engineering experiment in bacteria, you get visual results quickly. There is no such thing as cancer in bacteria: Solitary and rapid growth and division are without negative aspect in these unicellular organisms; there is no community to be disrupted.

Animal (and plant) cells are far different. They are hard to culture, fussy eaters, and often take days to divide rather than minutes. It is their inheritance to live in a community with other cells. They depend on other cells and other cell systems for nutrients, for signals that tell them when to grow and others that tell them when to stop; finally, they depend on other signals, often derived through physical contact, to tell them "where they are." Although these signals are still not well understood, scientists speculate that since all cells of an organism carry the same total complement of genetic information, these external signals must play a large role in determining whether a cell differentiates into a skin cell, a muscle cell, or a white blood cell.

On arriving at MIT, Land set to work to overcome the difficulties in culturing normal animal cells, and then to transform them by adding an oncogene to their own genes. The immortalized fibroblasts of NIH3t3 cells had already been transformed, so Land felt he had the best chance of success using cells of that tissue; the embryos of all animals grow explosively fast, so fibroblasts taken from rat embryos offered further possibilities. However, like those trying to transform the NIH3t3 cells years before him, Land had no luck transforming the fibroblasts for many months after his arrival.

Ras was known to be a potent oncogene; it was, after all, the one found in the human bladder cancer, and the retrovirus in which it had been found caused cancer in many animals; further, it was now known that ras was the oncogene that had transformed the NIH3t3 cells into a cancerous state in the Weinberg–Shih experiments.

A series of ideas and lucky accidents began to point the way for Land. Weinberg recalls that just about the time Land arrived, Weinberg attended a conference at M.D. Anderson in Houston, where one of the speakers was discussing two other investigators' work. A type of virus called polyoma causes cancer in mouse cells, but only under very special circumstances; these investigators had found that in order for it to transform cells, two oncogenes had to be active. The fact had no relevance to any of Weinberg's work at the time, but he tucked it away in his mind.

Further, work then-recently published by Weinberg's own lab

had shown there were two oncogenes present in several human leukemias. After months of failure at transforming fibroblasts with single oncogenes, therefore, Land set out on the far more difficult task of building two-oncogene units to insert into the fibroblast cells, using random combinations of the known cancer-causing genes.

Parada recalls that his own part in the scheme arose somewhat serendipitously. He had wanted to work with an oncogene called *myc*, and he talks about his desire to get hold of some the way auto enthusiasts might discuss wanting to put a rare, high-performance car through its paces.

"I kind of worked a trade with Bob [Weinberg]," he says. "He wanted me to hurry and finish a project I was working on, and he said if I did, he'd get me some *myc*." Parada adds with a mischievous grin, "I actually already had the *myc*; I was waiting for a chance to work on it."

Parada had become expert at gene cloning—getting a high number of copies and purifying gene-bearing DNA—through his work on the homology of *ras* and the human bladder cancer oncogene. He suggested that Land try *myc* and *ras* together to see if they could cause transformation, and he cloned the genes for Land to use. Land carried out the difficult transfections that yielded what, in this early summer of 1984, was the latest major breakthrough in Weinberg's lab: The *myc* and *ras* oncogenes in tandem were sufficient to transform an ordinary cell. *Myc* was an unusual choice, because the oncogene then had been found only in chicken tumors, but once the combination proved successful, characteristics of the two genes pointed the direction for further investigation. At almost the same time as the Land–Parada discovery, *myc* was found activated in the chromosomal translocation of Burkitt's lymphoma—that is, pieces of two chromosomes had been found swapped in this human cancer, and the result was to put the *myc* oncogene into a place where it would be activated.

Although their presence as oncogenes in viruses is limited, the normal counterparts of the *myc* and *ras* genes are found in nearly all animals. In fact, *ras* is so fundamental that it or a near relative is found even in such primitive microorganisms as yeast. Because the gene is so "strongly conserved" throughout living species, scientists are fairly sure that *ras*'s function is vital even though they don't know precisely what its protein does.

Ras encodes for a protein that circulates in the cytoplasm of the cell, the cellular "soup" between the outer membrane and the nucleus. *Myc*, meanwhile, encodes for a protein in the nucleus. This suggested that to cause transformation in ordinary cells, it might be necessary to have a combination of oncogenes that involve both cytoplasm and nucleus. Further, the *myc* oncogene appeared to confer immortality on the cell, while *ras* completed its transformation into the cancer type. This would explain why only *ras* was needed to transform the NIH3t3 cells, which already were immortalized. Much of this explanation was and is speculative, but now at last there was a certain ground to stand on: Normal cells had been transformed (following the rules set forth on p. 47) merely by the addition of oncogenes.

Since Land's two-gene transformation, he has continued on the same path: looking for new combinations of oncogenes. That is the aim of the experiment he is designing this afternoon, a warm one at the end of June. He is sitting at the bench and leafing through one of the innumerable blue-cloth three-ringed binders stacked or strewn throughout all the laboratories, the universal lab notebook, really a recipe book containing more precise versions of pinches of this and teaspoons of that. There is something just that basic about molecular biology labs, and something equally down-to-earth about most of the scientists who populate them. Despite the abstraction of the work and concepts—the invisibility of that world, the frequent difficulty in connecting the concepts to the reality of cancer—these scientists are on the whole a very practical-minded, physical, hands-on bunch.

Over one of the benches a radio is set to WBCN, "the rock of Boston," which prides itself on playing the latest and best of rock 'n' roll, as do many of the night clubs in Cambridge and Boston. Taped up on a bench, an eighteen-year-old front page from the *Baltimore Sun* proclaims the Orioles the world champions. The talk, the chatter, is far more often of what the Red Sox will do or of the investigators' own sports than of, say, art or what used to be called "longhair" music. Parada once said jokingly, "I have bad hands; I'm not that good in the lab. I'm really an idea man." That that athletic concept is used in these labs—and it often is—says something about the mindset of those who work here.

Politics: not surprisingly, generally liberal. Clothing: determinedly casual; jeans, coveralls, sneakers, sandals okay. Paula Traktman, former graduate student with David Baltimore and a good friend of Land and Parada, recalled, "I used to be considered very dressed going in to the lab. I don't mean dressed *up*, I mean I put on a dress." Beards and mustaches are common, haircuts infrequent. "Boats are okay," Paula says. "Sail, not power; wood, not fiberglass." There is also a distinct aversion to "gizmos."

There is a certain amount of high-tech equipment in a molecular biology lab, say an ultracentrifuge that might cost $30,000, or more recently, a gene synthesizer that will actually take inserted DNA bases and in hours (instead of months or years) assemble ten or more of the ordered sequence of bases, the code letters, to eventually form the desired gene. And some of the work in a modern laboratory is carried out with samples kept under glass hoods. The appearance is of protection for the experimenter; most often, scientists say, the hoods are used to protect the delicate laboratory-reared organisms from the virulent beasts that populate the air. The labs themselves are designed to contain whatever microbes are in use, but again, equally if not more so, to keep out foreign microbes.

This concession to high-tech aside, Land has an attitude common to basic science: "The ideal machine has three buttons," he says, "and that includes on and off. Too much of this stuff is too sophisticated; it gets between you and the thing itself."

Another scientist commented: "So many discoveries are the result of serendipity. Computers don't understand serendipity." Hands on, though what we are handling can't be handled and what we finally "see" is unseeable. The point remains, and it's a valid one: Discerning reality is the goal; nature must be played as closely as possible. Nothing fancy.

The Southern blot analysis, mentioned earlier as one of the most important techniques of molecular biology, is carried out using Seal-a-Meal bags from Sears and blotting paper not terribly different from the kind used to soak up ink. The pressure needed to compress the paper in a Southern blot is about five pounds. "I generally use a brick," Traktman says. Parada's homology experiments made him expert in doing Southern blots, bad hands aside. The "gels" that experimenters constantly "run" to differentiate proteins and different lengths of genes are carried out using equipment invented by molecular biologists from parts that cost under $30. The equipment is generally as simple as it is functional.

One lab is like another: a giant room sectioned by black-topped benches with see-through shelves containing bottles ranging from the mundane alcohol and water to the exotic fetal calf serum used as nutrient; tris, a buffer that keeps solutions from getting either too acidic or too alkaline; reagents marked with felt pen on labels of masking tape. The cabinets of blond wood are full of jars, and helter-skelter across the bench tops are plastic racks whose upturned fingers hold drying plastic test tubes; all around are boxes of Reynolds Wrap and Saran Wrap. In the next room are the vacuum hoods under which Land will do his transfections. Out in the hall are the "warm rooms" where cells are incubated, and in the lab are a couple of refrigerators with graffiti and clippings taped to the door.

As in any business, the personalization of the sterile workplace tells something of those who work here. On the refrigerator a note: "Tired of Molecular Biology?" And beneath it one newspaper ad for the CIA and another asking, "Where should you look for an exciting future in electronic warfare?" Mixed among everything else, on blackboards, on scattered slips of paper, the workers' notes to themselves and one another, sketched, crossed out: lines and circles that have been smacked by a (hopefully) masterly stroke of the felt-tipped pen to note where a string of DNA is to be cleaved, all done in the hieroglyphics of molecular genetics: BamHI, EcoRI.

In the popular imagination, the scientist is supposed to go to the board and write equations, and that probably is not the wrong image in some of the sciences. But not here; when molecular biologists think on paper or blackboard it is with drawings of schematic genes (straight lines), plasmids (circles, for these are little rings of DNA, of which more soon) slashed with designated "restriction" enzymes, enzymes that cut the DNA at specific base sites. There is EcoRI, "E-co R one," source *E. coli* strain RY13; BamHI, "Bam H one," source *Bacillus amyloliquefaciens*. There are the two restriction enzymes derived from the bacterium *Haemophilus aegyptius,* called HaeII and HaeIII, and the far better known derivative of *Haemophilus influenzae* strain Rd, called HindII, "Hin-dee-two."

On the wall next to Land a cartoon scientist, as shaggily bearded and long-haired as he, works feverishly with his test tubes over a caption that proclaims: "After considerable research Dr. [scrawled in] Land has discovered that the cause of cancer is the RATS THEM-SELVES!" Another artifact!

The simplicity and the functionalism all point up a major quality of these laboratories, and this may extend to other sciences as well but is nowhere more obvious: The only difference between various molecular biology laboratories is in the people who work there. If this seems to belabor a small point, it is a major point to the scientists themselves, and this particular laboratory has qualities that everyone agrees are unique. Here on the fifth floor, three of the country's most prominent molecular biologists work: Philip Sharp, an expert in gene regulation; Nobel Prize-winner David Baltimore; and Weinberg. The Baltimore and Weinberg labs are in fact mixed together, so that although the two men carry on different investigations and do not actually collaborate, there is constant interaction and conversation between their graduate students and postdoctoral fellows.

Land calls this "a very rare atmosphere, probably second to none, anywhere." And Parada points out that the way scientists learn to do experiments is from other scientists. "You come in, and you don't know how to go about things. I certainly didn't. So you ask and people tell you. It might be someone from Weinberg's lab or Baltimore's lab, and at first you might not even know which. You learn; you pass it along."

Land noted that social interaction thus is extremely important in molecular biology, and others in many different labs would repeatedly make similar assertions: Bright young people can discover themselves under the right mentor, in the right atmosphere, or be forever stunted by getting off to a bad start. Another major factor is that when we think of a working scientist, we tend to envision people of the ages of Weinberg and Baltimore—both in their forties. But in fact they are in charge of the laboratories; they do not actually conduct experiments. The bench scientists whose names account for the vast majority on scientific papers are graduate and postdoctoral students—people generally between twenty-two and thirty years old. They are selected by the man or woman in charge.

In choosing new people for the lab, Weinberg says, "I look for bright people, for intelligence. I don't care about specific techniques they might know; those they can learn as they need them. They have to be inquisitive and smart. And they have to be nice people"— underscoring the importance of this social interaction. "I won't take someone who's a pain in the ass, no matter how smart they are. It just doesn't work out in the long run."

Weinberg and Baltimore are both well liked by those in their labs, who virtually all share a fierce loyalty to their mentors and their groups, although those who run laboratories certainly are not universally beloved. The same kinds of gripes can be heard about other "lab bosses" as are heard of managers in any field: This one is a dictator; that one stands for no contradiction; another is mercurial, running through mood swings that keep the lab in total disarray; still another takes all the credit for work done by protégés.

All this is very much on the mind of everyone here these days, because soon "the fifth floor" will be history. Diagonally across the street from the cancer center rises the nicely designed Whitehead Institute for Biomedical Research, cause of considerable controversy when proposed a few years ago, now a reality. In a few short weeks, at the end of July 1984, Weinberg and Baltimore will move into new labs there, a monstrous job of logistics. Already boxes appear in the hallways here bearing cryptic labels, and notes on the bulletin board from the secretary who is the honcho for the operation warn of what will happen to those who do not follow schedules and procedures. The new facilities are beautiful, the equipment terrific, the space well designed, but no one is completely sure if it will really be the same, if the magic will keep working, if the god Serendipity will still shine down on them.

The other distinguishing feature of academic science, compared to that practiced in industry, is the constant turnover of people. Graduate students usually remain for four or five years, postdocs for one to three years. The only constant is the "lab boss," whose name is first on the door and, most often, last on the papers that come out of the lab—last because, like the director's name at the end of movie credits, it marks the person in charge of the work, overseeing, criticizing, suggesting, and finally approving; the preceding names tell who did the work and, often, who had the idea to begin with.

As a result, there is a certain amount of magic in these discoveries: the right mix of people, the right intellectual ferment, the right range of abilities—and then with serendipity, the answer falls out of the folds. But only, it seems, when you've done everything just right do you get this gift for the diligent.

Magical or not, this work is terrifically abstract. It is hard to get past the first step without having to pinch yourself: Is this cancer we're talking about? Or is it a laboratory artifact? Luis Parada himself suggests that near coincidence has brought basic researchers whose primary interest is developmental biology together under the banner of cancer research. "Next year, [in Paris] I may well be doing exactly what I'm doing now, investigating just these same problems, but it may not be called cancer research—and strictly speaking, it isn't."

Parada and I are working our way through a twisting series of hallways, then through the fire door; take the metal stairway up one flight, down a short corridor to a small room—really a storeroom with metal shelves containing stores of reagents and supplies, but also the home of some of the lab's experimental animals. Set inauspiciously atop a cabinet are the cages, each the size and shape of a shoebox, clear plastic with a Styrofoam top. Inside each box scamper four tiny pink hairless mice, with alert ruby-red eyes and huge ears, their noses constantly aquiver, but perhaps only because of the newly arrived human smell.

These are so-called nude mice, bred especially for laboratory work, a breed that has proven invaluable in cancer and other disease research. These mice have deficient immune systems—they have little ability to fight off any type of infection. That means that researchers can test the results of their work with less chance that the effects of various carcinogens are being hidden by the mouse's immune attack on them.

Each of these mice has at least one large tumor bulging beneath the skin of its shoulder; several have one on each. Most of the tumors are nearly the size of the mouse's own head, yet the mice appear in no pain. "They're not, usually," Parada says. "These tumors form just beneath the skin, and they don't metastasize." And that, of course, is part of the problem: No one has yet been able to *induce* a tumor to metastasize, so it is still a matter of heated debate whether metastasis is genetic—caused by the action or misaction of one or more genes—or epigenetic, originating outside the genes.

"We measure the tumor growth over a period of days or weeks, depending on what it is we're looking for, and the mice are sacrificed before the tumors become painful." Parada, who considers himself a softy, "sacrifices" his mice by dropping them one by one into a jar of ether. They are knocked out instantly and die quickly, he says.

Biology labs can be rough on softies, though; one friend told of his initiation as a summer worker before his freshman year in college, during which he had to kill dozens of white rats by snapping their necks—also supposedly a painless method, but certainly one requiring more gritting of the teeth. By contrast, Cantley and others study cells that must not be disturbed by a sudden influx of adrenalin and other hormones that might be triggered by ether; they must sacrifice mice by decapitating them in a small guillotine, painless to the mice but considerably more bloody than Parada's method.

All this may seem downright inhumane; on the other hand, remember Koch's postulates: We need to inoculate the suspected agent into a suitable host, which in fact becomes infected; we need to re-isolate the agent, and this requires using living animals. It makes no difference whether the agent is influenza virus or oncogenes, the question remains the same: Is this an artifact, a fact about how some cells behave in Bob Weinberg's lab dishes, or is this part of the reality of cancer, of *in vivo* cancer, cancer in a living thing, as opposed to *in vitro* cancer?

Still, it's an odd word, sacrificed; a reminder that, after all these years, we are still reading the signs and entrails of animals and trying to divine in them a message for ourselves. And then wondering, even when we seem dead right, if in some crucial way we're dead wrong.

Parada points to another set of mouse cages. "Those are being kept around a lot longer than mine. Those are Shelly Bernstein's."

Weinberg had told me about him. "Isn't he looking for a metastasis gene?"

"Yes."

So here was the colony in which Bernstein hoped to test Weinberg's belief that, like proliferation before it, metastasis, too, had its origin within the genes.

Out into the sunshine of late afternoon in what was an old urban renewal area that now is in that odd transitional state such neighborhoods go through: old, rundown buildings and warehouses interspersed with gleaming new ones. Corporate headquarters of Polaroid. The Whitehead Institute rising aluminum and brick from the rubble of construction: plywood concrete-frames, broken mortar, plank walkways. This whole section of town, tucked in a curve in the Charles River so it is about equidistant from the Harvard Bridge and the farther-north Longfellow Bridge, lay fallow for more than a dozen years. Its old buildings had been condemned and many had been razed to make way for a truly massive federal project.

This corner of Cambridge was to be Mission Control Headquarters for NASA, so the story goes. Then the Massachusetts-born-and-bred President of the United States was assassinated, and the Texan who succeeded him decided that Mission Control would be in Houston, in the New West. So it went, so it goes; science, business, and politics have a long history together, ever rocky. And it is a history prominent with "swashbucklers," men who have seized the moment to make happen what they chose to happen. A frequently heard term in molecular biology as in medicine: Sidney Farber was a swashbuckler, Jack Whitehead is a swashbuckler. Swashbucklers don't follow the rules, they stir up trouble, make waves, just swashbuckle ahead; and they get things done. The bottom line: They get things done. Swashbuckler is not entirely a word of approbation but, like *macho*, there is a strong undercurrent of respect in it. Swashbucklers build such places as the Dana–Farber Cancer Institute, which can be seen from here although it is miles away in mid-Boston. Swashbucklers start building construction, according to popular legend, without waiting for the nicety of a building permit (that related by Emil Frei concerning Sidney Farber). And they build the Whitehead Institute for Biomedical Research after overcoming enormous initial opposition from MIT's faculty over control of the institute's faculty. And, of course, if either building is one day remembered as the place where the riddle of cancer was solved, where the Gordian Knot was either untied or cut (which will it turn out to be?), then the swashbucklers will have been right.

7

Small World

"Try telling this to someone who's sick: You have a mutation from glycine to valine in the twelfth amino acid of your *ras* gene. That's why you've got bladder cancer. I know that, but I can't do a damn thing for it. On the other hand, your doctor, who doesn't know what's going on in there, can do something for you."

Paula Traktman contemplates the gulf between basic science and the applications in the clinic as we sit on a park bench near her Cambridge apartment. An ethnic food festival is whirling around us, and it's a bright, blowing June day. "Still, those of us in basic science have a commitment to thinking that the more you know the better you'll be. In the long run," she says.

Traktman is a virologist, her current emphasis on the vaccinia virus, a relative of variola, the agent responsible for smallpox. In this small world of basic cancer research she has extraordinarily good ties. About to leave Cambridge for Cornell University Medical College in Manhattan, where she will be an assistant professor, she became a postdoctoral fellow with Bryan Roberts at Harvard Medical School after completing graduate studies with Baltimore, and considers Weinberg a friend and mentor. Although her own work did not directly involve the transformation experiments as the decade turned, she watched it all from up close. She was an undergraduate student of Lynn Klotz, whom she had only recently met again after several years, just as Lew Cantley was Klotz's junior colleague and Tom Roberts his postdoctoral student at Harvard. All of them eventually will figure in this story in very different ways.

It is Klotz who introduced me to all of them, who first related to me the common threads emerging in all that he has read and heard of cancer, that many once-unrelated causes and types of cancer were "coming down through a funnel of a few very fundamental concepts."

At the moment Traktman is reviewing the recent history of her field, a period that has seen sea changes in outlook. In some ways this seems strange to her: She, Weinberg, Baltimore, Land, Parada, all are very basic scientists; yet cancer research, if only because it is so practically oriented, is really applied science. "It's funny to have an army of basic biologists working on something that must be considered applied science," she says. "Ordinarily those of us in basic science have felt distant from applied science." She notes that funding agencies also draw sharp lines between basic and applied research. (Freireich's observations would come frequently to mind.)

Looking back, she sees as a major conceptual discovery the realization that certain retroviruses had captured cellular genes, had mutated these genes in the capture, and now could cause rapid cancerous transformation in hosts they infected. "This was the moment when we had in hand a proof of basic science. We realized that the way these viruses go about acquiring genes and becoming rapidly tumorigenic, mutating and altering their expression, is a mirror for what's going on in the human cancer. It also showed that there was a lot more unity in the world than skeptics had believed."

In fact, transforming viruses turned out to be divisible into two categories: those that had captured an oncogene and could rapidly transform cells they infected, and those that might lie dormant for years before causing transformation. These latter turned out to provide another vital bit of information about how cancer starts: They caused transformation when they accidentally inserted their powerful gene controls in front of a cellular gene that is normally quiet. They offered, in other words, yet another simple mirror for how cancer *in life* might begin.

And that is why, abstracted from the clinic as this scientific quest for the causes of cancer might be, explaining real, clinical cancer is still certainly the goal, and aiding in the curing of cancer certainly is a hope—however long-term the basic scientists' discoveries are in their usefulness.

So far there has been an exciting synergy in the molecular discoveries in many once barely related fields. For example, Traktman points out, while "the virologists had been characterizing the behavior of retroviruses, the classical people were characterizing the nature of the cancer cell." Each was of vital importance. For example, for Weinberg to know that indeed he had transformed a cell, whether with virus or chemical, he used "assays that the people studying cancer cells gave us," she says, referring to the tests outlined in chapter 1.

Like virology and cytology, "All the fields of cell biochemistry have come together under what would be called the study of molecular genetics."

But what remains to be learned is as vast as what has been found. "We have to find out what the oncogene product is doing," Traktman says. "To say that cancer results from the mis-action of a gene or genes is one thing; to know how the altered proteins function to cause transformation, and to know that all the further steps in oncogenesis are genetic, those are very different things."

And that leads me to an exasperated question (the exasperation not mine alone). When do we get to say, "That's it, there's the end of the road, the answer, the final spike in the last rail"? At what point, that is, could cancer be said to be understood?

"Maybe never."

Another fascinating analogy concerning polio. "We don't know why people get polio. We know how: A virus causes it. We also know that in 90 percent of the population, those who are infected get an undetectable stomach virus. In some relatively small proportion the virus climbs up the spinal column and causes paralysis, even death. Why? We don't know; thirty years after a vaccine was discovered that prevents it, we don't know."

There remains a strong association between viruses and cancer. As important as it was to look within the cell to find the true origin of the disease, the moment when it could truly be said to begin, viruses *or* environmental carcinogens can also play a role. For example, Burkitt's lymphoma is a cancer far more common in Equatorial Africa than in the rest of the world. Nearly all those afflicted with it are found to be infected with Epstein–Barr virus. Yet this is a common virus; in the United States, as in the rest of the West, it causes mononucleosis, endemic in college populations.

How can the same virus lead to a deadly cancer in one group, and to a serious but survivable sickness in another? No one knows. But most of those who develop Burkitt's lymphoma have also had malaria, and scientists speculate that the two may twist the right genetic combination for cancer. Similarly, liver cancer is widespread in the Third World, and at highest risk for it are those who have had hepatitis, the virally caused liver infection.

A virus called papilloma, long studied for its transformation of animal cells in the laboratory, is being increasingly implicated in uterine cancer in women. But notice that as we return to old notions, circling constantly, we don't come back to quite the same place. Papilloma doesn't simply *cause* uterine cancer, any more than hepatitis virus causes liver cancer or Epstein–Barr causes Burkitt's. In some relatively small percentage of the population, these viruses are doing something, presumably, to human genes. Some kind of genetic mis-action still seems to lie at the very foundation of the cancer process, its first step.

8

Oysters, Pearls

Weinberg is recounting the work of other scientists in providing background for the successful Land experiments in transformation. "There was first the work of Cuzin and Rassoulzadegan as reported by their co-collaborator Bob Kamen at an M. D. Anderson conference, and into these suggestions of two-oncogene action in cancerous transformation came the work of Van Der Eb in the Netherlands, who had shown two active oncogenes in adenovirus, and simultaneously his own awareness of multiple active oncogenes, specifically *myc* and *ras*, in several human leukemias. And the rest is history."

The rest? An ordinary conversation with Weinberg is much like a history lesson. His conversation has an unusual quality: not only does he speak in complete, grammatical sentences, but they are completely footnoted and referenced. (John Cairns, another molecular biologist of great repute with whom I spoke later in the summer, has that same characteristic.) Most people's sentences flow in straight lines; Weinberg's flow like growing trees, with parallel lines developing, converging, splitting. Maybe it is years spent addressing conferences, maybe he's accustomed to using a dictaphone, but it is not a trait I found in most other scientists. Ask about the work in Weinberg's own lab and invariably the description, lucid and logical, includes citation of the work in any of a half dozen other laboratories, including the spellings of investigators' names.

Equally distinctive is his ability to interrupt in midsentence—a sentence encompassing the march of all molecular biology toward oncogenes, a sentence of many clauses and citations—pick up a different conversation entirely, and resume with the word following his breakpoint. Noticeable when talking to him in person, the effect is most dramatic as I review an interview taped over lunch.

Setting: the seafood restaurant down the street from his lab (equidistant, in fact, from the old and the new laboratories). My wife, Ginny; son Daniel, seven; daughter Katie, five; Weinberg, and I are all in cross-conversation. Clatter of silverware, roar of lunch-hour conversations. Tortuous sentences concerning the scoring of foci of NIH3t3 cells are broken by the ubiquitous "Good afternoon, I'm so-and-so, and I'll be your waiter today."

And here's Weinberg at a critical point in time: "Now this homology between oncogenic sequences which had been thought entirely unrelated, between [the viral] Harvey's *ras* and the EJ human bladder oncogenes was demonstrated in the laboratory of Geoffrey Cooper of DFCI. . . . Would you like some dessert?" He leans forward, talking to the kids. "Your father says you don't like ice cream. Is that true?" Not true! On and on. Ice cream ordered, waiter gone, he resumes: ". . . as well as, of course, in our own laboratory through the work of graduate student Luis Parada, whom you know. . . ." And he proceeds onward as though the entire complex chain of statements, as though the answers to questions, sat ready inside his head, preformed.

We had wound up at lunch after he rushed in late from a weekend in New Hampshire, where he and his family own a small farm."Eaten alive by bugs," while spending the morning tying up tomato plants. It was now only two days before the Big Move. What is interesting about listening to the history of oncogene research according to Weinberg is that he never fails to mention either competitors or investigators in other fields whose work struck him. His narratives thus are not only complete, they agree note for note with those offered by scientists further removed from the story and therefore more dispassionate.

What is apparent from these branched-tree histories is that Weinberg's laboratory is one of the central stalks of the plant, the plant being the development of current theories of oncogenesis relative to the behavior of cancer genes. He didn't do everything, nor did his workers always get to press first, but somehow they did nearly everything; if they were not first in print, then they were in print with such solid information that it tended to establish other evidence. Barbacid himself said as much in recounting how his own group had published the first evidence that the *ras* viral and human bladder oncogenes were in fact one. And Parada recalled a feeling of exasperation when, after he had discovered the homology, "Bob had me do it and redo it and prove it eight ways. My God, by the time we published we had it nailed so solidly that no one could dispute it."

And, in fact, most people in the field remember the homology as having been reported out of Weinberg's lab, because he and Parada had announced their evidence to other scientists at a meeting in Squaw Valley. Who gets credit for what and how much credit is granted is no cut-and-dried affair in science. There is publication, but the quality and solidity of the experiments reported, as well as to what degree general claims can be made from the results, all account for the far more subtle yet most important ways that scientists judge one another.

And that points up an interesting quality in all the people whose names are brought up most frequently in the cancer gene story, whether Weinberg, Wigler, or Geoffrey Cooper. They all had reputations as good scientists, people who did solid work that could be trusted. But outside the confines of their own specialties, they were largely unknown. They were not "golden boys," young scientists of such obvious promise that even their odd-sounding ideas would be seriously considered. They were in a hot race for discovery, but they were really racing each other. Finally, when it came down to the race to isolate the oncogene causing transformation, Weinberg, Wigler, and Cooper all used considerably different stratagems to isolate it. They all succeeded, and thus each in turn offered confirmation of the others' work.

This thread of citation that runs throughout Weinberg's sentences is more than force of habit, it hints at much of his character. He never forgets where an idea came from; he never forgets where he came from or where any aspect of him originated. Hence the tale of his and George Khoury's trip to a Pittsburgh symposium, memorialized in a poster, the only decoration on Khoury's wall.

Weinberg was born in 1942 in a middle-class Pittsburgh neighborhood. The son of German immigrants, he spoke German at home and remembers starting Linden Elementary School with a German accent. At Linden his mathematics teacher was Margaret Maloney, and his science teacher was Sarah Schmeltz. Significance? George Khoury was Weinberg's classmate there. So was Frank Solomon, whose laboratory is just down the hall from Weinberg's. And Steve Lippard, MIT chemistry professor. And Jim Haber of Brandeis. Now, here are five top scientists engaged in some of the most advanced research in the country, and they have only one thing in common: They were taught elementaary science by Sarah Schmeltz and math by Margaret Maloney at Linden Elementary School in Pittsburgh, Pennsylvania. That doesn't mean there aren't more such scientists out there; but these five all know one another.

Weinberg and Khoury were invited to take part in a Pittsburgh symposium last spring, March '84, and agreed, provided they could be given one evening free. Granted. They looked up Miss Maloney and Miss Schmeltz, now both retired, and took them out to dinner. "We had a great time," Weinberg remembers.

What was so remarkable about the education they all had? Weinberg shrugs. "It was no one thing they taught us. They just gave us that feeling, from the very beginning, for a good education, for sound principles."

Nevertheless, it was no golden boy who set off for MIT hoping for a career in medicine. Weinberg's undergraduate career could serve as inspiration for young underachievers everywhere. For openers, he got a D in his first biology course. Then, although improved, the rest of his grades were "so mediocre that MIT was the only graduate school I could get into, because they knew me here, knew me as a person." Major universities generally follow a practice of not admitting their own undergraduates to graduate programs, to avoid inbreeding. Weinberg is an exception: "I am a product of total academic incest," he says—B.S. and Ph.D., and, finally, tenured full professor, all at the same university. Weinberg spent one year teaching at Stillman College in Tuscaloosa, Alabama, a year's postdoctoral fellowship at Israel's Weizmann Institute, and another year and a half as a postdoc with Renato Dulbecco at the Salk Institute in La

Jolla, California. Except for that relatively brief period, Weinberg has been at MIT since 1960.

Paula Traktman sums Weinberg up in a word: "Rabbinical." And watching him precisely articulate the steps from present to past, past to present, forward and back and forward again, whether his own personal history or that of his science, it is an apt description. He cuts loose no threads: still speaks fluently the German of his childhood; speaks Hebrew. It is perfectly in character that he has traced his family tree as a hobby and named his son Aron, after an ancestor he traced to Napoleonic Europe. Weinberg, wife Amy, daughter Leah Rosa, and son now live in the Boston suburb of Brookline, where he regularly leads Passover seders, hosting colleagues and students.

And now, forward: "I have in my mind a complete picture of how the cancer process occurs, a model for how each step might occur. This is based largely on the work of others, in smaller part on my own imagination; I am convinced it works that way." Pause. "Of course, my conviction may not carry much weight with the Almighty."

Later that afternoon I am in Lew Cantley's lab at Harvard. His blackboard is covered with chemical scrawls; calcium ions float past sodium ions, strange alphabet-soup concoctions degrade into everstranger ones. Cantley's own work is not focused directly on oncogenes, but it is cancer-related, and he has followed the cancer-gene story with intense interest. A highly articulate scientist with an extraordinarily orderly mind, Cantley is now trying to put in perspective the accomplishments of Weinberg, Wigler, Cooper, Barbacid, and the others prominent in unraveling this first-step story.

Orderly mind: "There are three categories of experiments you can do," says Cantley, an associate professor in the department of biochemistry and molecular biology here. "I teach all my students to evaluate every experiment they do according to what category it falls into.

"Category I are questions that will be answered yes or no by the experiment you've designed, and either yes or no will tell you something. Are the odds of the experiment's working better than 50–50? Then go; either answer advances knowledge.

"Category II experiments are those in which a 'yes' answer to your question tells you something, a 'no' tells you nothing. 'No' just means the experiment didn't work; the gene didn't express itself, whatever; you don't know why. If the odds of this one working are about 50–50, you're in the category good scientists spend most of their time working in.

"And finally, there's category III: Only a yes answer will tell you anything, and the odds that you'll get an answer are less than 50–50. If I'm right on a category III, I've made a major advance; if I'm wrong, I've just wasted my time.

"The key point is, students have to decide: How much time is worth the risk? If you're proposing a category III experiment, how long will it take? Would you spend two years on it? A really interesting question to me is: Were these Weinberg experiments category III? He certainly had to believe he was going to get his answer to keep going through those initial transactions; he had to believe. A 'no transformation' answer there is useless, and there was no evidence that he would get transformation, so the odds had to be well under 50–50 at that point.

"But here's the thing: Every good scientist invests something of himself in those category III experiments. They're the ones that push you forward, push your whole field forward. But how much time and energy do you have the nerve to invest?"

Cantley pointed out that Weinberg, Cooper, and Wigler only a few years ago were not universally applauded. "Theirs were all small labs, not the kind of big lab where you could take major risks more easily. And they persevered in the face of some very strong criticism."

It would have been all the more interesting a commentary had I known then, as I learned later in the summer, that the hieroglyphics on Cantley's blackboard contained what Cantley believes is a chunk of the answer Weinberg was speculating on over lunch: the missing links in cancer-gene explanation. What do oncogenes do? That is, what do their proteins *do* in a cell? Ray Erikson of Harvard had begun to pry that answer loose, discovering a key enzyme activity for the protein product of the *src* oncogene—the oncogene of Rous sarcoma virus. Cantley had teamed up with Erikson on one important recent experiment. Right now he was collaborating with Dana–Farber's Tom Roberts, one of the country's leading experts at getting genes to overexpress themselves (to produce large quantities of protein). They would prove what Cantley now already firmly believed: that at least some oncogenes sharply affect the activities of an important group of intracellular molecules called second messengers. More of that later, as it happened. The key word, perhaps the champion tongue-twister of this story:

phosphatidylinositol

It becomes first sayable, then as unforgettable as a radio jingle, when sung out with proper attention to meter:

PHOS-pha-TI-dyl in-OS-i-tol

A song in iambic quatrimeter.

9

The Real World

Remember looking inside the animal cages as Luis Parada measured the swellings: Beneath their pale pink skin, the mice had tumors of which they seemed hardly aware but that were real nonetheless, palpable, measurable. The tumors were nonmetastatic, so you could not go so far as to say those nude mice had cancer. But with the injection into them of cells that had undergone the action only of oncogenes named *myc* and *ras*, those mice had grown tumorous masses.

Ancient conundrums have their way of looping back forever. What is real: the abstract world of ideas (The Real) or the concrete here and now (the real)? When you press into reductionism in science, there's no escaping the sense you are in the realm of Ideas—despite the principal aim of explaining complex ideas with simpler ones. When that complex idea is cancer and we are lost in this maze of steps and progressions, these ideas seem more creatures of the brain than concrete objects. But yielding to this dichotomy in what is real is quite contrary to the idea of modern science. The idea of science and its temple, the laboratory, is to fuse those two notions into one.

The idea of the laboratory is not very old, and abstraction lies at its heart. Galileo and his circle generally are credited with creating the laboratory as a model of the real world, and that only about

350 years ago, a short time when compared to the many millennia-old ideas in science, mathematics, and medicine. The Greeks, for all their great ability at abstract thinking, tried to study and explain natural forces out in the "real world." To learn about friction, they observed sailors dragging ships from ocean to beach. Conversely, they tried to intuit natural laws by purely abstract reasoning, which worked well enough (some say) in Euclidean geometry but not in physics or biology. It has been pointed out that Aristotle, considered the father of biology, continued to propagate the popular myth that women have fewer teeth than men, when all he had to do to establish the truth was to count them.

So if the idea of the laboratory involves the idea of abstracting the real, equally importantly it involves *realizing*, concretizing, the abstract. The experiment is observation, but it is fully controlled, prepared observation.

That was the Galilean idea: to build a model, an abstract of the real world in which the force or principle under investigation could be studied in isolation. Conversely again, the model would be a realization, a concrete example of an abstract concept that allowed you to articulate it. It did indeed represent a fusion of the hard-rock idea of reality and the abstract idea of Reality, a fusion at work through the whole of the Renaissance in every endeavor. Artists studied anatomy and mathematics side by side with scientists, were now and then the same in the person of a Leonardo da Vinci.

But make no mistake, the clinic—especially the clinic of a teaching hospital—is as good an example of this Renaissance laboratory as is the virologist's lab. The two, in fact, nicely define two ends of a spectrum: the clinic where cancer comes in the door; the virology lab where the most vital concepts and "things" are not seeable at all.

Walking down a Cambridge street, late July 3, heading toward the MIT cancer research center. The music of rock bars bounces out, reflects around the streets. The street musicians are already working Harvard Square, jugglers, magicians thick among the evening strollers. A local rock singer, Joanne Cipolla, has just finished a song at Jak's that she wrote, and it has been clattering in my head, a song called "Vanishing Species." She sings of the dead species of the world, the brontosaur and pterodactyl, and some day *you may awake and find you're vanishing, too!* But the end is most intriguing: *and then there are all the children, all the kids you played with when you were little—whatever happened to them? Where did they go?*

Vanished, in a way, but not as a species; nearly everything but. The line set this hurried-up movie running in my mind: Here we were, small children, our cells dividing into new daughter cells as replacements for dying cells. By the time we reached adulthood, virtually every cell in our bodies had been replaced, except for fully developed brain nerve cells and a few others, which are added to as we grow, but not replaced. Vanished!

Even more dramatically, consider yourself a brand-new adult of eighteen, containing the ten trillion cells of an adult and looking just like yourself. The John/Jane Doe Colony. Ten years after this "snapshot," how much of you is left? Red blood cells are programmed to die in about one hundred days. The vital epithelial cells—the layer that generates new cells of skin and the inner linings of most organs, including the digestive system—similarly turn over every few months, but some cells of the colon and the blood-forming bone marrow last only hours. Even the long-lived cells of the liver die in less than two years. Watch yourself as a moving picture now, hurrying through time: a full-grown man or woman, vanishing before your own eyes (which are vanishing too). Left are the neural cells of the brain, which from adulthood onward are never added to. But at least we can see most of the brain moving onward in time, a single entity, as the rest of the body fades and disappears a little each day.

What's left? But that's easy: The Plan remains. The plan for you remains clicking along in ten trillion nearly identical copies, one copy per cell, to be passed along to each of the new cells whose generation it dictates. The whole plan, strung out in a chain six feet long, is packed up in submicroscopic skeins of chromosomes, slipped into the microscopic nucleus of a minuscule cell.

Do you believe that?

10

Midnight Oil

Monday I'll do the paperwork for the experiment, decide how much of what is needed, how long the experiment should run, the logistics. Tuesday night I'll precipitate the cells with DNA, and on Wednesday check the cells. The cells have to be left with the calcium phosphate for seven to ten hours.

The night had just rolled into the morning of the Fourth of July when Huki Land began the final stage of this round of experiments, experiments aimed at finding pairs of oncogenes that would transform normal cells. Now he sits at his transfection bench, before the clear-glass sliding door of the vented hood, inside which are the tools of his trade: dozens of little covered plastic dishes containing liquids that resemble rosé wine. We onlookers sit on either side of him, the other visitor being a French scientist who is interested in learning the techniques Land developed and described in his paper on the cooperation between *myc* and *ras* in transforming cells. He is here because there is no substitute for seeing the experiment done, possibly picking up on little tricks that might make all the difference.

Tonight is the culmination of two weeks' work, but the results won't be known for another two; and therein lies much of the difficulty of working in mammalian cell systems: What bacteria or viruses might disclose overnight can take a month in these higher organisms, starting with preparation of the cultures. Last week Land prepared his rat-embryo fibroblast cells, sacrificing a pregnant rat, removing fibroblast tissue from the embryo, placing the fibroblast in solution with collagenase. Collagenase is an enzyme that will later be seen as an important target in the development of malignancy; here it is used to break the cells free of the tough microscopic webbing of the protein collagen that holds them together.

We tend to think of connective tissue as meaning ligament or cartilage exclusively, but the term refers to a tissue type virtually universal in the body. Most animal cells have the consistency of bags of jelly. Unlike plant cells, they have no tough outer cellulose wall to make each unit stiff. But these individual little sacks are plugged solidly into a meshlike network, known as the extracellular matrix, by certain surface receptors. This matrix is formed largely of collagen, one of the toughest proteins there is; the pattern of the collagen framework is responsible for much of the "architecture" of tissues. Collagen*ase* is an enzyme that dissolves collagen; it is used in some meat tenderizers. Land uses it to free the embryonic fibroblast cells to grow them in culture.

"We'd like to take a cancer gene and put it in a normal, epithelial bladder cell," he says. "The problem is that in culture those cells grow poorly, and they take up DNA poorly, so our experimental system has to be simpler. We use embryo fibroblasts from rats, but they're not immortalized. They'll grow ten to twenty generations and then die. It's normal tissue, but it's still experimental, an *in vitro* model."

So there is one side of the experiment: developing the primary culture of normal cells in which Land will attempt to induce transformation. On the other side, he has his elaborately crafted oncogene mechanism. Tonight he will attempt to get the oncogenes into the DNA of fibroblast cells. Oncogenes, we now know, are normal cellular genes that for one of a variety of reasons have begun working improperly, coding for altered proteins or coding for the right proteins at the wrong time. Land has spent the past week building "machinery" he hopes will get the oncogenes to express themselves —translate into protein—once they are inside the cells he's cultured, that is, incorporated into the normal complement of DNA. Unlike the cells, which could be seen under any microscope, the genetic machinery is of that Never-Never-Land below vision, but here is how we imagine it.

By now the image of cellular DNA has been invoked regularly: the super-long, double-coiled thread of genetic instructions for building a living thing. It is very difficult to work with because of its length, compounded in higher organisms by its being packed into chromosomes. Bacterial DNA is simpler and therefore offers a better system for growing up genes. Many bacteria, as noted, reproduce every twenty minutes; that means they duplicate their own genes that frequently. Through the techniques of genetic engineering, scientists have learned to insert foreign genes into bacteria—human or other mammalian genes they want to grow up in large quantity for study. Thus, every time the bacteria divide, they reproduce the foreign DNA along with their own, and every time the bacterial DNA is translated into proteins, the foreign genes are likewise expressed.

When scientists talk of cloning genes, they are referring to the often arduous process of growing up large numbers of a gene of interest that may be present in a given cell only in one or two copies; that one or two copies might be sufficient, as in the case of the original transfection experiments, to make a "normal" NIH3t3 cell cancerous; but given the dimensions of a single gene, it is hardly big enough to study. Millions of copies of the gene are needed for study. Growing the gene up in bacteria is the way to get those copies; and even better, there are tiny circles of DNA called plasmids that are relatively easy to work with, and that inject themselves into bacteria.

Plasmid rings are tiny even in relation to a bacterium's gene complement. For some reason, in addition to their cellular DNA, bacteria often carry supplemental genetic information in the form of these small plasmid rings. The rings frequently are passed among bacteria, conferring on them special abilities and defenses that may be needed in particular environments. These plasmids may contain as few as two or three genes, and that means an oncogene can be inserted into one without fear of its getting lost in the genetic jungle. Land has inserted his oncogene pairs into plasmids, then mixed the plasmids into a colony of bacteria.

Only ten years ago themselves the objects of the most advanced scientific study, plasmids now are "built to suit" by biological supply

houses and supplied to researchers by the jar. Also available for pur-
chase are enzymes of a bewildering variety: the aforementioned restriction enzyme that will snip open a plasmid ring at a specific base
sequence, another that will cut any DNA chain at every place a
particular base sequence occurs to break the molecule into, say, gene-
sized fragments. Other restriction enzymes have the effect of making
the ends of plasmid DNA segments "sticky" so they will reanneal into
rings.

The result of all this submolecular tool-building is that Land can
snip open plasmid DNA rings, insert one or two oncogenes, insert
mechanisms called promoters and enhancers, which help the genes
express themselves, seal the rings back up, then put the plasmids into
bacteria. He will grow a large colony of those bacteria, break open
the cells, and remove the bacterial and genetically engineered plasmid
DNA.

The final step is fairly simple. By late last week, Land had a jar of
thick, mucus-like liquid containing this raw bacterial and plasmid
DNA mixed together. The liquid has that consistency because the
DNA is so long and has been grown up in such quantity it makes its
medium extremely viscous.

In fact, DNA is so long relative to its width that if you don't
care how big the fragments are (as Land does not in this experiment),
you can break the molecule by squirting it through a fine glass pipette.
The sheer force alone will shatter the molecule into thousands of segments. The fact was more of a shock to biochemists than it would
be to a layman; never before had scientists run into a strongly
bonded chemical compound that could be broken by sheer force.
The idea seemed as far out as hacking at water with a meat cleaver
and expecting to get hydrogen and oxygen.

Now Land had to separate the bacterial DNA from the plasmid
DNA in his jar, because the plasmid DNA contained the oncogones;
this separation is simple because the DNA lengths vary radically. The
bacterial DNA clings to the bacterial-cell debris, forming a heavier
mass that can be spun down in a centrifuge, leaving the lighter
plasmid DNA at the top. The plasmids then are separated out of the
liquid by putting them in a chemical "gradient"—a liquid more
dense at the bottom than at the top; the plasmids will form a distinctive band at the appropriate density level and can be removed.

To complete Land's preparations, he had to get the plasmids out of their solution, so he added any one of a variety of chemicals that caused them to precipitate to the bottom of their tubes, then he added alcohol to wash off the extraneous materials. So he begins tonight with two sets of ingredients. First, he has cells taken from rat embryos, connective tissue cells that have now been incubating in their primary culture for nearly a week; these cells will divide only a few times on their own, because that's how their genetic instructions program them to behave. Second, he has plasmids-bearing oncogenes in a solution of alcohol. In the silent, otherwise deserted laboratories, the only sound other than our conversation is the whirring of two vacuum pumps: one under the hood, creating an inner airflow to separate the experiment from the experimenter, and one Land is using to suck ethanol off the plasmids.

This is fairly tedious, routine work. There are probably well over one hundred dishes here, each containing various combinations of oncogenes; included tonight are the oncogenes *erbB* and *myb*. There are duplicate dishes for each combination.

"These cells are nowhere as good as NIH3t3 at taking up [foreign] DNA," Land says. In that established cell line, in a given volume of cells, five thousand might take up DNA, offering a good chance that the oncogene pairs would at least make their way into the cells. But in these normal fibroblast cells, which have not been immortalized, in the same volume only three hundred cells will take up DNA at all, even with the inducements Land is using.

Now he adds calcium phosphate to the mixture; this is the special gimmick in a family recipe, discovered by scientists in the Netherlands in the early 1970s. In solution, the calcium half of calcium phosphate has a very strong positive electrical charge. DNA has a negative charge, which is part of the reason DNA will not pass through the outer membrane of a mammalian cell. Somehow, in ways not yet entirely understood, the presence of the added calcium ion neutralizes the DNA so that more cells will admit it through their membranes. Although the percentage is still extremely tiny, it is a large enough number to offer hope that over the range of quantities in the experiment, any potent oncogene combination will function, if not as well as *myc* and *ras*, at least well enough to be detected.

By function, Land notes, he doesn't mean transform every cell the oncogenes manage to enter. "Even *ras* and *myc* in combination won't do that, though we're not sure why. There could be a third element needed for a cell to have sensitivity to the action of the other two."

So what we three are looking at here, through the hood's glass, as though watching TV, is the pouring of rosé-colored waters from dish to dish. And what we hope we're witnessing is this: The cells are growing on the surface of the lab dishes, and you can imagine them blown up like giant soap bubbles side by side; they need the contact of the dish in order to grow. When they grow large enough, each will split into two growing bubbles, then four. Now relatively tiny plasmids begin to drift slowly down, many settling on the filmy cell membranes, and now the presence of calcium with its double-positive charge enables some few of these filaments to slip through the membranes to vanish into the cells' interior. The coloration is from phenol red, a marker whose color varies to show the pH or acid-base concentration; rosé is just the right color for these cells.

"Is the time between adding the calcium phosphate to the DNA and putting the DNA on the cells critical?" the French visitor asks.

"No," Land says. "It's only important that the precipitate [of DNA] doesn't turn to concrete. Then it is very hard to work with."

He is now "plating" the cells. With a calibrated pipette he draws up a particular quantity of fibroblast cell–DNA mix and squirts it into a waiting lab dish to which nutrient has been added. On and on, carrying stacks of ten or twenty finished lab dishes to the incubator, where they will be maintained at body temperature for the next few weeks. As he plates the cells, he swirls the mixture in a series of broken, irregular motions, as though he were panning for gold in these tiny dishes, and comments, "You have to be very careful you don't introduce regular motion into the dishes" when plating. Such regular motion might cause the cells to settle in a regular pattern—such as concentric rings or another wave-sedimentation pattern —that would yield false readings in the resulting cultures.

"Most of this is very routine," Land says. "Of course, if you screw it up, there goes two weeks' work. And there's always the competition. Losing two weeks could prove very costly. That's another kind of pressure added on." It's a difficult kind of pressure, because most of what is being done here cannot be speeded up; therefore the pressure must be dealt with while waiting, keeping busy doing something else until results show or enough time passes that you can conclude they aren't going to.

The problem with this kind of experiment, Land notes, is that negative results will be meaningless. In this case, so many things can go wrong that learning that oncogenes A and B do not transform cells might mean only that the experiment was not designed right. Land has taken great pains, on the other hand, to make sure that a positive result will mean that they do transform in tandem, to make sure that such a result would not be artifactual.

A variety of steps can be taken in an experiment to safeguard against false readings, chief among which are using positive and negative controls. Imagine a hypothetical experiment using both. We have a plasmid containing oncogenes A and B, which we can call plasmid (A+B). The experimental question is, are these sufficient to transform a normal cell into a cancerous one? We have defined our criteria for "cancerous" as carefully as possible and built the experiment to follow those criteria: Perhaps we are going to see if the cells expressing (A+B) will grow in soft agar, the near-liquid nutrient in which normal cells will not grow, or will grow foci, or will form tumors in nude mice; perhaps all three.

Land tonight is using a positive control. Along with the experimental gene pairs he is using the *myc–ras* combination that he had already found to be so potent. We know these will transform cells. Even if (A+B) do not enable cells to form foci, those dishes containing (*myc+ras*) should. If this does *not* happen, then there is something wrong with our experimental system; and that's why we're doing it. The positive control, in other words, should work even if the oncogenes under study do not. A negative control might involve using a single-gene system that should *not* cause transformation; if transformation occurs, again that shows a flaw in the experimental system.

There is another feature of this experiment that is common in molecular biology laboratories these days, especially those involved in cancer research: This is not a quantitative experiment but a qualitative one. To be sure, Land measures out his ingredients, watches temperatures and acid–base concentrations, but the results, he notes, will be visual ones. He will see the dark stars of transformation or he will not. The nude mice will grow tumors or they will not. How quickly and in what quantity these things happen is of secondary importance; the real question is whether they happen at all.

It is well past 2:30 A.M. on the Fourth of July before Land finishes plating his cells. He will be back in the morning to separate out the calcium phosphate, seven to ten hours after they were mixed.

11

The Clinic

Shelly Bernstein is intense. That is not the first impression he makes, but once the realization takes hold it is reflected in his every movement. He is about thirty, has a wiry build and fine features, black curly hair, and a black mustache. He wanted to be a doctor "for as long as I can remember," and he is one, and almost as soon as he was introduced to pediatric oncology he knew that was the area he would concentrate in. By the time he mentions that his old schedule was rough—"I would go in [to the hospital] at seven or eight in the morning and come home at nine or ten at night, mentally and emotionally exhausted, but I enjoyed it"—it is not a surprise; he seems the sort of person who would work such a schedule and find in it a certain exhilaration.

Intense: his words are calm and measured, assured and reassuring regardless of the subject, qualities no doubt important to the bedside manner of a doctor dealing constantly with children and their parents, and with children seriously ill, whom he sometimes loses. This morning he has only two patients, so there is time to talk here in his office at Boston's Dana–Farber Cancer Institute.

Bernstein has both an M.D. and Ph.D., a combination indicating his dual interests in clinical medicine and research, although none of his research experience was as basic as that he's done in the past year, as a visiting scientist in Robert Weinberg's laboratory at MIT and the Whitehead Institute. Now he wears two hats, spends some mornings here at the clinic, afternoons across the river at the lab; yet despite the very different sets of demands on him, he finds his schedule lighter than it had been when he was a clinical fellow.

Bernstein became interested in genetics as an undergraduate, extended that interest in medical school to the genetics of a human disorder: sickle cell anemia. He became so absorbed by this often fatal blood disorder most common in blacks that he interrupted his medical studies to work on his Ph.D. for a year in Cameroon, Africa, between 1976 and 1977. "It was an interesting, memorable year for me in Africa," he says.

He returned to finish his work on both degrees and decided to specialize in pediatrics, but it would not be general pediatrics. "I love kids and I love seeing healthy kids, but I'd rather take care of a very sick patient that had the potential for being cured, albeit small, and become intimately involved with the patient and his family." Bernstein specialized in pediatric hematology—the branch of medicine concerned with blood disorders—at nearby Children's Hospital and continued concentrating on sickle cell anemia. But there were many cancer patients at Children's, and it was not long before the treatment of cancer in children became his overriding passion.

"In general pediatrics, you might see a patient every six months to a year and never really get to know them," he says. "Here, I often see patients every week, sometimes twice a week, and you develop a very close relationship with the whole family. After their hospitalization, they're usually in regularly as outpatients. We're on a first-name basis. Every day of their lives is affected by what I decide: They need to know whether they can go out in the sun because of their chemotherapy, whether they can go to camp. It's often a frightening thought, how dependent they really are, but it's a major responsibility I enjoy, being that involved and being able to do something good."

Bernstein notes that it was not many years ago that childhood cancer was usually incurable. The statistics have changed radically. More than 50 percent of all childhood cancers now can be cured— at least, the children are surviving past the five-year period statisticians use to determine survival rates. Much of that improvement owes to the work of Emil Freireich and Emil "Tom" Frei, whose office is on the tenth floor here. The improvement came from new chemotherapy techniques. Although the basis of chemotherapy has never changed, the amounts and types of drugs used have changed considerably over the forty-plus years since nitrogen mustard was found effective against certain cancers.

Chemotherapy has proven especially effective against leukemia, and leukemia accounts for more than half of all childhood cancers, with 85 percent being of the form called acute lymphocytic leukemia (ALL).

All chemotherapy drugs are toxins, a fact that some critics have used to ridicule the practice, calling medical oncologists "poison doctors." Frei himself says he loses his composure at such talk. The drugs kill cells, but not indiscriminately. They kill the fastest-growing cells preferentially, and that means they kill more cancer cells than normal cells. That is the basis of chemotherapy, which can be administered systemically, to strike at tumors that may have metastasized. Radiation kills all cells, but it can be very finely targeted. So the majority of modern cancer treatment involves surgery to remove the visible tumor or tumors, irradiation to kill whatever tumor cells may have been missed in the surgery, then chemotherapy, called adjuvant chemotherapy when administered in conjunction with other treatments to strike at farther spread cells.

Nevertheless, some of these drug regimens are so toxic that patients die of their side effects, and radiation therapy has been strongly implicated in causing later cancers in some of those who are treated with it. But these most radical regimens are used only against the most certainly fatal forms of cancer.

All chemotherapy drugs so far found kill other rapidly growing cells as well as tumor cells, and chief among these are epithelial cells: cells of the stomach lining, subsurface skin cells, hair follicle cells. The result is intense nausea, vomiting, and sometimes diarrhea for hours after the drug injection, and usually complete hair loss. The hair loss is, fortunately, temporary, but it's often psychologically devastating to cancer victims, especially teenagers whose self-images are already shaken by their disease. The parents of child cancer victims say other children sometimes ridicule them for their baldness. In recent years, hair loss has been prevented in some patients by having them wear "cold caps," which make the hair follicle cells

sluggish and slow to divide, preventing their being killed in chemotherapy treatment.

There are two explanations for the nausea that follows chemotherapy, each steadfastly defended by its own group of doctors. One
is that killing the epithelial cells of the stomach lining produces the
nausea; the other is that the toxins act on the vomit-center in the
brain, where the nervous system takes emergency reflexive action
against anything registering there as a poison, forcing it to be dis-
charged. Those arguing the latter explanation point out that people
being given chemotherapy begin to throw up virtually instantane-
ously, too fast for it to be the result of cells being sloughed off,
which might take hours. On the other hand, as another physician
noted, some chemotherapeutic agents never pass the blood–brain
barrier—never get to the vomit center—but cause vomiting as intense
as others that do. Whichever is true, the speed of the reaction is not
disputed, and those who have had chemotherapy, adults or children,
say that if new regimens could be found to eliminate nausea then
chemotherapy would hold no dread for them. A great deal of work
has focused on that problem, with some success reported lately.

The speed and certainty of patients' reactions to chemotherapy
drugs unfortunately was not known to the Dana–Farber Cancer
Institute's interior designers. Oncologists entering the sparkling new
building for the first time were alarmed: The entire lobby was covered
in bright red carpet, the intention presumably to help create a cheerful atmosphere. Unfortunately, the carpet perfectly matched the
color of Adriamycin, an antibiotic discovered in 1967 that has become
one of the major chemotherapy drugs. The doctors' warnings went
unheeded until so many patients had thrown up reflexively on entering the lobby that the carpet was replaced; it's now neutrally beige.

Plants are the source of most anti-cancer toxins, developed evolu-
tionarily, it is supposed, to ward off predators: An animal getting
sick from eating a plant would not likely return to it. Ricin, a common drug in several protocols, comes from the castor bean; vinca
alkaloids like vincristine and vinblastine come from the periwinkle
plant. Antibiotics, like Adriamycin, are produced by bacteria to ward
off other bacteria. The actions of most of these drugs involve combination or interference with nucleic acids, either the DNA itself or
one of its related molecules. Some drugs prevent the DNA from

replicating so the cell cannot reproduce. Others simply stop the DNA from being properly expressed, to yield proteins needed for its cell's life.

Despite this general knowledge, Tom Frei noted, the reasons why some drugs work are quite often not known. The first evidence that nitrogen mustard might work followed the World War I battle of Ypres, where thousands of soldiers were gassed. Later a group of investigators discovered that rats died after eating vincas, and that the particular action of something in the plants was to shut off white cell production. Those were serendipitous discoveries. "Finding new drugs is a mix of scientific investigation, empiricism [screening potential drugs by trial and error], and serendipity," Frei says. "But the key is always observation by a prepared and active mind."

Frei has been an oncologist long enough to see a sea change in both treatment and, even more significantly, attitude toward cancer. "Thirty years ago the attitude of many doctors was that there was no point in working in cancer; there was nothing you could do. When I was at NCI, I was told by many people, go into basic research, that's the only way cancer can be taken care of." Yet by 1970 children with ALL were being cured by the regimen he helped develop. Upwards of half of childhood ALL cases are now permanently cured. The success, he says, is the result of the integration of basic and clinical research, but it took no small amount of courage for early medical practitioners to take the first steps in chemotherapy: "These were toxic drugs, and basically scientists were saying they wouldn't work."

The public attitude toward cancer has changed too, Frei says, all for the better. Years ago, cancer meant death, stigma, and pain. Like tuberculosis in the nineteenth century, it was a plague simply to be avoided. Now the disease is "out of the closet—it's just another disease, to be faced." And part of that is because it can be cured, he says. "We can cure half the people who walk in the door; there are a lot more that we can help"—extending their lives often by years— "and we are learning to manage the side effects [of the treatment]."

By contrast, in the past the vast majority of cancer patients were not even told what they had. "This completely broke the integrity of the relationship between doctor and patient," Frei says. "It left the patient isolated from both doctor and family; that was all wrong.

Even now we don't tell patients everything at the first sitting, but we do eventually try to tell them the whole story. We do level with them. If we fail we tell them." Frei noted that the 50-percent cure rate is misleading in two ways: once-deadly testicular cancer is now 90 percent curable, while the most severe lung cancers and cancers of the liver and pancreas are still virtually incurable, so the average does not offer a true picture of how a particular cancer responds to treatment.

That leads in turn to another question, put to George Canellos, Dana–Farber's chief of medical oncology: What about those who cannot be cured? How does one learn to deal with the knowledge that many people will die? Canellos, his British accent authoritative, replied, "Sometimes the hardest thing for a doctor to do is to do nothing. The younger the doctor, the more that is true. They come here, out of medical school, convinced they can save everyone. And they confront a patient who pleads, 'Help me, doctor!' And suddenly they confront the fact that there is nothing they can do, no treatment. That is very hard to accept, but of course they have to accept it."

And Craig Henderson, chief of the institute's breast cancer clinic: "A doctor has to realize he does something by his presence, that his presence and willingness to listen are often all that he can give, but they are important."

Tacked up on Bernstein's bulletin board is the Dana–Farber newsletter. Two children smile down from a page-one photo, flanked by two staff people. Both children are very round-faced, moon-faced, and the girl wears a turban. She is Jacquelyn Manzi, Bernstein's first patient today; the boy is Patrick Gormely, who will be in in a few days. Jacquelyn's face is still quite round, a temporary condition caused by prednisone, a steroid that is part of her chemotherapy treatment. (Steroids act on molecules that bind to DNA, affecting cellular reproduction.) But she is obviously a pretty girl, just turned eighteen, having come through a storm few adults have faced.

The second youngest of six children, Jacquelyn began complaining of leg cramps to her mother, Anne, a nurse. "She wasn't eating right, and we were concerned that she had anorexia. She just had no appetite," Anne Manzi remembers. "She was pale and fatigued." The diagnosis took no time: her white blood count had soared and other major blood factors were skewed. She had ALL, the most common childhood leukemia, rare in adults. Jacquelyn remembers the period right after her treatment began as the worst. In the ward, "We all looked the same: no hair, round faces, puffy eyes." The day after she entered the hospital, a boy about her age was admitted, also suffering from ALL. They became good friends, and she regularly inquires about him.

Both were discovered to have chromosomal translocations, always found in a different type of leukemia but rare in this one. In fact, Bernstein noted, he has seen only two ALL patients with such translocations, and they entered this hospital a day apart, an amazing coincidence.

Recent discoveries concerning chromosomal translocations offered major new evidence supporting those who believed the actions of oncogenes were the cause of human cancers. As mentioned before, the DNA of higher animals is packed into chromosomes, like wool in a skein. Humans have forty-six chromosomes: twenty-two pairs of similar chromosomes, which scientists simply number consecutively, plus an X and a Y chromosome for men or two X chromosomes for women. One set of twenty-two plus the sex-determining chromosome are inherited from each parent. This means that although in any given pair the two chromosomes are not identical, the same characteristics will be found in the same location on each. That is, every gene has an "address," a precise location on one chromosome. But in a translocation, a piece of one chromosome winds up on another, and in some cases pieces of chromosomes can actually be exchanged.

Both Jacquelyn Manzi and her friend had a part of chromosome 4 translocated onto chromosome 11. The effect of a translocation can be serious, since the regulation of gene expression is vitally important to cell growth. Some genes are expected to turn on regularly, to mount immune responses to viral attacks, for example, or to replenish dead blood cells. Several years ago, Michael Cole, then of Washington University in St. Louis, discovered that a long-known translocation in Burkitt's lymphoma resulted in the *myc* oncogene being placed directly in front of the controls for the immunoglobulin gene, which makes that protein so important to the body's immune response. This was an exciting finding. The immunoglobulin gene must be frequently expressed, so here was yet another picture of how an oncogene might do its work: It might be a normal gene that had somehow come under the regulation of "hot" controls, so that it was constantly expressed, instead of rarely.

In many ways the most important result of the discovery of the oncogene in that translocation, Weinberg had noted, was that for the first time a phenomenon visible under the light microscope (translocation) had been matched with invisible phenomena (oncogene expression) until then detectable only in the laboratory. Since then, several other translocations have been discovered, although it is not yet proven that they *cause* cancer. They are associated with some cancers; correlation is not cause. It is still not known what effect the 4–11 chromosomal translocation has.

Anne Manzi relates how devastated the family was when they learned Jacquelyn had cancer. Her hospital roommate was in worse condition, having just had a bone marrow transplant for advanced Hodgkin's disease, and Jacquelyn cried that if the girl died it meant she too would die. The girl died within days. Then Jacquelyn had a severe reaction to L-asparaginase, a chemotherapy drug. It caused bleeding in her brain that made her weak on one side, as though she had had a stroke. She was taken off the drug, then later put back on it and carefully monitored. This time she had no bad reactions, went quickly into remission, and has remained apparently free of cancer for some eighteen months now. In April 1985, she would be taken off her chemotherapy—two years from the date of her remission.

Remission is a difficult state for oncologists to assess. It means that there is no sign of cancer. In the case of tumorous cancers, cancer is nearly always undetectable until the tumor grows to about a billion cells, a mass of about two centimeters in diameter. Some cannot be detected until they are even larger. Bernstein explained, "We assume that between surgery [for operable tumors], chemotherapy, and radiation we've reduced the cancerous cells to a low enough level that the immune system can clean up the remainder." In other words, doctors do not assume that in remission all the cancerous cells are dead. In fact, evidence from chemotherapy indicates that a drug always kills a given *percentage* of tumor cells, not a given number; thus subsequent drug treatments cut tumor size by a percentage—which mathematically may approach but never equal zero. So, "for the duration of remission," he says, "we assume that the remaining cells have indeed been killed by the immune system; but we never know that." Chemotherapy continues for a predetermined period, in this case two years. And epidemiologists assume that any tumor that has not returned or metastasized within five years is in fact gone—although this is certainly not always the case.

Bernstein takes Jacquelyn into the examining room behind his office, and her mother comments, "We've had a lot of financial troubles, and now they're worse." Her husband, Frank, is a maintenance worker with the housing authority in Webster, where they live, but even on their two salaries cancer is not affordable. Returning, Bernstein says she "continues to do well," looking now at her chart. There has been no sign of a relapse since she went into remission, and she is pleased that her treatment is to end in months. Her hair has grown back in, still fairly short but stylishly so, dark brown and curly. Before chemotherapy it was straight, she says, and Bernstein adds that a change in hair texture is common, though no one is sure why it occurs.

The visit is brief, once every three weeks, though Jacquelyn takes medication at home. Her chemotherapy will be administered here by a nurse.

John Cabral will have to stay longer, by only half an hour, but it is a half-hour he hates. Today the eleven-year-old boy has to have a bone-marrow sample taken and, although he gets a local anesthetic before the long marrow-drawing needle is inserted, he cries out in pain for the perhaps ten seconds it takes Bernstein to press it into his hip and withdraw it again. Throughout, Bernstein speaks in a voice that is gentle but authoritative, explaining each move he makes, and it is all over with quick precision.

"All done," he says. "John always finds this especially painful."

John had come in with his mother, Aldina, who emigrated from the Portuguese Azores when the boy was only thirteen months old. He is the youngest of five children, and the whole family has been having a rough time since he got cancer. Aldina and John's father have been separated for several years. She and the children had been camping at Lake George, New York, when John fell ill with fever; he couldn't sleep and his breathing was difficult. Aldina took him to a hospital in Framingham, where they live, and was referred to Boston Children's. An x-ray disclosed a tumor mass in the boy's chest, and a biopsy of his lymph nodes showed it was ALL. That was two years ago, before he was ten. That and other indicators put John out of the high-risk group. He has been treated with vincristine and methotrexate, another common chemotherapy drug, but two weeks ago suffered cramps and stomachache. Bernstein does not think that is serious but wants to continue monitoring his condition.

"John likes to paint, he's very active," Aldina says. "But his brothers and sisters don't understand. Sometimes they have a rough time with him. He throws temper tantrums and they don't understand what's wrong, and they see him getting a lot of attention." She shows wallet pictures of all her children, the oldest nineteen, then John as a small boy with a thin rather than round face, wide-eyed and curious. She dreams of taking John back to the Azores one day so he can see where he was born.

His prognosis is also good. He has been apparently free of cancer for nearly two years now and is to begin fifth grade in the fall. He lies on the hospital gurney, encircled by nurses and his mother, relieved but not smiling as the marrow sample is taken away for analysis. Under a microscope, a technician will look for any sign that white blood cell production has gone awry.

We are walking through the clinic now, a place made as cheerful as possible. Next to it is a ward-style room containing rows of beds and easy chairs; children come here in the afternoon for chemotherapy, stay several hours with their parents, and go home in the evenings. The schedule can put families through harrowing rearrangements of their lives. Steve Woodcheke and his wife, Nancy, are at the front counter with their three daughters. Amy, the eldest, has ALL, but in her it progressed so far she had to have a bone marrow transplant. It began when she was two years old; suddenly she stopped walking. For months, her pediatrician said there was nothing wrong, though she cried a great deal; then he said it was arthritis and wanted to put her on aspirin therapy. The Woodchekes took the girl to a rheumatologist, who suspected leukemia; she suspected Amy wasn't walking because she was suffering hairline bone fractures that were causing her pain.

Amy was finally diagnosed at the Jewish Hospital Center on Long

Island, where the family lives. She went into remission immediately and remained so for two-and-a-half years, then relapsed. The family, who had hoped their agony was ended, was stunned. Amy was referred here for her bone marrow transplant in August 1983. She remained hospitalized until October. Her mother, pregnant with the couple's third child, stayed in Boston. Neighbors helped, caring for the remaining daughter. For the year since then, Amy has been fine.

Bone marrow transplants are the most severe of the therapies for leukemia, and children who reach the stage of needing one often do not survive. The transplant, as Bernstein explained, is not really the therapy, it is the rescue. The therapy is to so irradiate the body that all the bone marrow cells are killed, cancerous or not. Then new bone marrow is implanted to begin producing the white blood cells vital to the immune response. Until they begin working, for many weeks, patients must remain in 100 percent sterile environments, eating sterilized food, communicating with all visitors only by telephone. There is also a strong danger of rejection of the new marrow, as there is with any transplant. In some cases a small amount of the patient's own marrow, known to be free of cancer cells, can be removed before the irradiation and then replaced, lessening the risk of rejection; this is known as an autologous transplant. When that is not possible, allogenic transplants are done (literally from the same species, but donors generally have to be close relatives for there to even be a hope of matching marrow types).

The Woodchekes are up from Long Island for a bone marrow check now, waiting to see Amy's doctor. Around the waiting room are plastered letters and pictures that show the range of ages of the patients in this unit, from the cheerful scrawls of toddlers to fine drawings by high-school-age children. Letters of thanks, birthday cards to doctors, newspaper clippings telling of the courage of young patients from here in carrying out school activities. A plaque shows a smiling Charlie Brown with the adage: "God made some heads perfect. The rest he covered with hair." A few steps down the hall is where the Monday afternoon clinical conferences are held.

The medical staff of pediatric oncology sits around a large conference table. The chief of the pediatric staff, the nursing director, pharmacologist, doctors are here to discuss current cases, especially those with problems. One doctor reports a problem with a patient— really with the patient's father—over an upcoming transplant. The doctors will hash out, sometimes argue over, the course of therapy being given, the way results are interpreted, or the prognosis; the chief of staff is quick to question and challenge assertions.

Bernstein, who sits at the opposite end of the table from him, is reporting one case for another physician who is absent, the case of a girl who had been doing beautifully, then died suddenly of massive bleeding. He also has a case of his own to present, that of Patrick Gormely, who had had Hodgkin's disease with involvement of the right cervical nodes for four months. This is an optimistic report with little comment or question: Gormely seems to be doing fine.

Not so in June 1983.

Patrick Gormely, twelve and a half, fifth-grader, lives in North Hampton with his mother, Sandra, a nurse in an acute head-injury clinic. His father, Richard, is a police officer in nearby Carlisle; works the four-to-midnight shift, so he could be here today too. Parents are separated. When Patrick complained of cramps and tiredness a year ago, the family doctor dismissed the symptoms. Sandra was furious that tests had not been done. She took Patrick to nearby Denton Cooley hospital, where he was found to have a swelling in the right side of his neck. An X-ray showed a tumor mass in his chest about the size of his heart and nodules on his lungs, a sign of spreading that immediately classified him as Stage IV Hodgkin's disease.

The Gormelys agree that she, with her medical background, was the more devastated by the diagnosis. "I was hysterical," Sandra says. "I think it's worse if you're trained and you know what to expect." Richard adds, "That's true. I didn't really know what any of it meant. I was worried, but I didn't really know what they were talking about. From then on, of course, I read every book I could get my hands on."

Patrick was put on a chemotherapy regimen including nitrogen mustard for six months. There were a lot of ups and downs. On the up side, doctors had scheduled him for surgery for a biopsy at one point. Ten minutes before surgery was scheduled, an X-ray showed the tumor mass completely gone. But then Patrick suffered from shingles, commonly seen in children with Hodgkin's disease. Bernstein says that more than half the children who have had chicken pox get shingles, which is caused by the same virus, because their immune systems are depressed. Patrick was in excruciating pain from the shingles and was put on codeine. He has scars all over his chest from the shingles, his mother says.

It was he who was photographed with Jacquelyn Manzi in the hospital newsletter, his face also round and his body plump from chemotherapy, which often causes water retention in patients. He was given Torecan, an antinausea drug, but one that had a rare side effect that Bernstein calls scary: It occasionally causes patients to shake and stare blankly into space. These side effects were easily reversed with another drug, Benadryl. Patrick still tires easily, though this summer he went to a camp at Lake Winnipesaukee, New Hampshire, run just for children with cancer and free of charge. He looks as healthy and happy now as any boy, blond-haired and freckled, quick to smile, the roundness gone from his face, although his mother says he has had an upset stomach the past few days. But Bernstein says his progress appears good; he is to return in three months for another checkup. The one negative that remains is warts: Patrick has had large-scale eruptions of them. Virally caused, they too imply a depression of the immune system that ought to be combatting them.

Bernstein is in the x-ray room now, a narrow, dark corridor whose walls are entirely illuminated, translucent, so that X-rays can be posted and read. He is pointing to the area of Patrick's chest where the tumor had been, now believed clear; but to be sure he calls to a radiologist standing nearby and asks him to confirm his reading. He does so. And then there is more time to talk.

Bernstein started in Weinberg's lab a year earlier, and here there was a fortuitous meeting of the minds. As a clinical oncologist, Bernstein naturally had a deep interest in metastasis, the killer in virtually all cancer, and the leukemia he saw most often was systemic in virtually all cases. He arrived at just about the time Weinberg was seeking someone interested in testing his own belief that a gene—at least a small number of genes—was responsible for this ultimate step. Bernstein had been seeking a research post where he could study the molecular biology of cancer, because for all his general background in genetics he had never done molecular biology before.

His mentor at Dana–Farber found several possibilities, but Bernstein simply felt he and Weinberg hit it off well: "I felt completely comfortable; it clicked." Neither he nor Weinberg was specifically thinking of the metastasis experiments when Bernstein was picked, both say; that was a lucky coincidence that came later.

Bernstein admits to some rough times when he first arrived, going from being an experienced, expert physician to a beginner in an advanced molecular biology laboratory. "I suddenly felt completely wet behind the ears, on the bottom rung, like the lowest of grad students or even an undergrad." Bernstein actually was better off than many M.D.s; he had had advanced laboratory work to earn his Ph.D. He had kept up his reading in *Science* and *Nature*, the latter of which he says latched on the most quickly to the oncogene story and therefore got the cream of the papers in the field. When he knew he was coming to Weinberg's lab he began reading *Cell*, which he feels is the very best in the specialized areas of molecular biology and oncogenes. Most doctors do not read basic research journals like *Cell*, any more than the molecular biologists read *JAMA* (the *Journal of the American Medical Association*) or *Hospital Practice*. There is some crossover, Bernstein says, with such magazines as *Nature* and *Science* read by both groups. And of course there is *The New England Journal of Medicine*, the most prestigious of U.S. science-medical journals.

If it took Bernstein a while to get his feet on the ground at MIT, he says others in the lab made the going fast. He began by tackling oncogene transfections and Southern blots, "the bread-and-butter techniques of Weinberg's lab." Now he has a colony of several hundred mice in a couple of different locations, and his basic aim has been to cause benign tumors in the mice to become metastatic by inserting genes into the tumor cells.

He brings a thorough knowledge of clinical cancer—cancer the human killer—into the laboratory, a perspective few others in this lab have. Not all labs are so clearly dedicated to basic research. Bernstein's wife is a Ph.D. researcher at Harvard Medical School, and in her lab, which is run by an M.D., there are people doing clinical as well as basic research.

But, he is asked, isn't the recent excitement in the field caused by the dovetailing of separate views of cancer? As though common roots had been found for totally different languages, the speech of Babel suddenly seen unified and singular more than divergent?

"I think so, I hope so. And that's what I hope I've brought, is the clinical perspective. It can be a serious problem in any basic lab. People know molecular biology perfectly well but have never seen a cancer patient, unless it's been by accident. When we talk metastasis or the idea of benign versus malignant, they know what happens in a cell, by definition. But they have no clinical conception of a patient, and that's what I hope I add."

Bernstein theoretically works full time in Weinberg's lab, but he returns for his Monday clinic, and he keeps in regular contact with all his hospitalized patients. He even still maintains a hematology clinic a couple of times a month at Children's Hospital. Last night, he spent an hour and a half here when one of two patients he had been following closely relapsed. "I can't ignore my patients," he says. "I had to talk to the parents, to decide what to do. I usually visit the hospital in the morning or swing by at night on my way home. Any major decisions that need to be made are mine."

On the other hand, "They don't bug me across the [Charles] River for minor 'housekeeping chores.' Many doctors are obliged to handle those things because they're close by." And he says although life is intense during his hospital and clinic visits, "It used to be that way every day for me. . . . But I enjoyed it very much, it was so challenging; that's what shifted me from hematology."

12

Roller Coaster

Crossing the Charles River Dam bridge from Cambridge to Boston, you drop down onto the city shore just before it fans out into the harbor's Atlantic seascape, not far from the mouth of the river. And right at the doorway of the Boston Science Museum, a fascinating collection of machines to work and gizmos to light up to illustrate a world of scientific principles. A laboratory in a certain sense? It would indeed be a laboratory if those who built these wondrous constructs were not sure what the machines would do when they were set in motion. If they had built them, that is, to show themselves how energy was transferred, how waves moved, how light split into its component colors, or how electric bolts of electricity could snap between the poles of a Van de Graaff generator, then this would be a laboratory. But they built these devices to show us what they already knew, so it is both fascinating and instructive, but it is not *doing* science. There is no investigation, no uncertainty, no chilly fog of ignorance (hopefully about to burn off in a dazzling burst of light).

The device that seems to absorb most people's interest looks like a small roller coaster, complete with a loop and some high banked turns, upgrades, plunges. You start by launching a softball-sized metallic ball at the top, and an illuminated digital counter tells you how much energy the ball has. It is kinetic energy, the energy of motion, but it can be translated back and forth into other types of energy. Much of the biological life process involves such translation, so few things are more vital than how the transfer of energy occurs and how it is controlled.

The ball starts with potential energy based on the vertical height it will fall during its tortuous descent, and with kinetic energy based on the impulse the player delivers to launch it on its way.

Descending, the kinetic energy rises, the ball picks up speed as that potential energy of gravity force is converted into kinetic energy. Then it rounds a sharp curve and loses energy, transmitting it into the tracks: that is the energy required to change it out of its straight-line travel. A lot of the energy—probably most—is lost to friction, given off as heat. Now the loop-the-loop and a big drop in energy (kinetic changed to potential as it goes up in the air) followed by a regain (potential changed to kinetic as it descends). It never regains all it lost, of course: Some energy was needed for that change in direction from straight line to circular, and much is lost to friction. Now it slams into a line of four identical balls ahead of it in the track, and it comes to a complete halt. The lead ball takes off in its stead, registering kinetic energy it got from the impulse transmitted, springlike, through the chain of balls (minus some energy lost in between). This lead ball now gains some kinetic energy (converted from its potential, based on its height as it began), loses some on an upturn, loses some more as it sets in motion a line of swinging rods (their motion energized to the degree the ball lost energy), and finally "punches in" its remaining energy figure at the bottom, ending up with zero kinetic energy.

The key point of his energy transfer, of course, is that all these little bits of energy add up, right on the nose. The amount lost to friction, the amounts transferred to each object, converted into potential energy with each rise and back into kinetic energy of motion, and finally the amount of energy delivered at the bottom add up exactly to the amount of energy the ball started with. Nothing is lost; nothing is gained. Energy is conserved.

In the world we live in, not needing to be Einsteinian unless we're talking about atomic reactions or near-light speed, energy is *always* conserved. That is true in any human body at any given moment. Food carries energy packed in the bonds of the molecules that make it up. When we digest the food, the molecules are broken down into simpler molecules, a downhill chemical reaction, and energy is made available. When we carry out any activity, such as flexing our fingers, energy is demanded: a downhill chemical reaction to fuel an uphill mechanical reaction.

Energy release is largely carried out by oxidation. Put a flame to wood with plenty of oxygen available from air, and the wood oxidizes: It burns. At the end you get ashes—oxidized wood—a collection of molecules at a much lower (downhill) energy state than the original wood. The difference in energy is given off as heat and light. Expose iron to air and the iron oxidizes; look across a rusting junkyard and you're watching metal burn, a slow burn to the eye but burning just the same, its molecules combining with oxygen to form lower-energy-state iron oxides, rust. Quite appropriately, energywise the junkyard is headed downhill.

Problem: Wood, coal, and other fuels give off their enormous quantities of stored energy to combustion at high temperatures, temperatures at which flesh and bone would combust as well, temperatures far beyond the tolerance of living things. On the other hand, although iron rusts at air temperature, it oxidizes far too slowly to provide the quantity of energy needed by a muscle called upon to contract explosively. So how does a living system constantly, with every sleeping breath and beat of the heart, with every sudden tiger's spring, run this incredibly complex roller coaster of energy transfer?

Nature solved that problem with a remarkable chemical device called the catalyst. A catalyst is a molecule that enables two other molecules to join together or split apart using far less energy than would ordinarily be required. In effect this means that a chemical reaction that might occur ordinarily with near-zero frequency can be made to occur any time its catalyst is present. Enzymes are nothing more than biological catalysts; they are proteins that mediate chemical reactions in living things, permitting such reactions as oxidation to occur rapidly and frequently at the narrow "temperature window" within which life exists.

It is something of a corollary of the rules of evolution that when nature solves a problem, that solution tends to be repeated over and over again throughout the living world, and that is nowhere more apparent than in enzyme catalysis. Chemical reactions always involve the loss or gain of energy (They are downhill or uphill). Virtually every chemical reaction in every living organism on earth is mediated by an enzyme, generally one unique enzyme for each chemical reaction. Thousands of distinctly different enzymes are at work in the human body at one time or another, some operating virtually continuously, others used only for specific purposes and so operating intermittently, still others used extremely rarely.

It's hard to overstate the importance of enzymes to life's processes. James Watson noted, "Enzymes effectively determine the chemical reactions that occur in the cell." And that is the key to enzymes' importance, a heritage of that narrow window of temperatures within which life nestles. The reactions within living things *ordinarily* would not occur within the temperature range in which life exists; therefore we can call up precisely the reactions we want in the order and frequency we want them simply by controlling which enzymes are present and in what quantity at any given time.

Toss a log on a fire and see spontaneous oxidation taking place, but only at high temperature; watch a tree grow and see the equally powerful opposite chemical reaction taking place to store that enormous quantity of energy, a reaction taking place at air temperature via the mediation of enzymes.

Where is all this leading us? Hopefully straight and true to the target: The molecular biologist's attack on cancer is based on the idea of reductionism. A complex idea can be understood by breaking it down into its simpler components, then understanding each component. A physical process, no matter how complex, can be understood by breaking it down into its component actions and understanding each of them. It is reductionism that claims the topsy-turvy motions of the steel ball on the roller coaster can be comprehended by breaking those motions, those energy transfers, down into particular components and explaining them. We have no doubt in the twentieth century that such reductionism is possible in explaining mechanics and energy transfer, though it was doubted quite steadfastly in Galileo's time; but reductionism is a controversial notion and perhaps always will be when human life becomes a focus of its practitioners. There is a very similar dispute in cancer research between basic scientists, who always seek to *reduce* such processes as malignancy to a series of precisely definable physical events, and those who see in such disease indefinable qualities that can only be attacked head on, at the level of life at which they occur.

This opposition to reductionism can take many radically different forms. Reconsider the "conquest" of polio. Paula Traktman pointed out that although Salk discovered a means of stimulating the body's defenses against this virus, in a reductionist sense we still don't understand it at all. And in another range, there are large numbers of people, some physicians among them, who subscribe to a "holistic" idea of the cause, cure, and prevention of cancer and other diseases: Cancer is a disease "caused" by the whole human going out of whack, and conscious effort on the human's part can restore health. Many reputable people believe this, and many former cancer victims swear they have been cured by following prescriptions based on a holistic rather than a reductionist view of health.

I offer no argument against them. I have no cure for cancer nor do I know of anyone who does. But something interesting happened in the intellectual life of the West within the last few decades, and cancer has much to do with it. Cancer, as I pointed out earlier, has become a system of its own. It has become a place that scientists go to understand life, just as surely as it has become a scourge to be conquered. And in that sense of understanding, we are talking of reductionism, no mistaking it. Striking the target dead center may or may not lift the scourge of cancer, but it certainly will provide understanding. Scientists are after knowledge when they study cancer—clean, precise, step-by-step, clear knowledge with no yawning chasms, as there surely are right now.

Back to enzymes. We are looking at cancer as a physical process within the body. One cell grows when it should not, divides into two when it should not; in the ultimate step, tumor cells uproot from their matrix base, their anchorage, and drift to far corners of the body where they continue to grow in an environment that should be hostile to them, but is not. Reactions and more reactions, tall hills up and down, great loops of energy transfers, and that means enzymatic proteins determining those reactions, and in the growth of the tumor mass we see billions of cells being built out of structural proteins.

Tumors develop their own blood supplies, needing vast amounts of blood's oxygen energy for their growth. Tumors are powerhouses.

One means of locating breast tumors too small to feel is to take a thermogram, a temperature scan of the breast; for tumors form hot spots, spewing energy in far greater amounts than normal cells.

* * *

Where else can that lead us but back, deep within the cell to the nucleus and within the nucleus to the master tape coding for every last one of those proteins, enzymatic or structural: the jungle of 100,000 genes, the intervening DNA sequences with often mysterious purpose, and material packing the DNA twine into chromosome rods. How does it work? What does "code" mean in this context? What does it mean for a gene to be on or off, and just how is a gene read out?

Back in the darkness of the mental theater, let's change the way we build the DNA now to reflect some of its other features. The result will still look like a spiral staircase, more or less. Each of the bases, A, T, G, and C in the DNA double helix, is attached to a sugar-phosphate backbone. This backbone forms the sides of the spiral ladder, while the bases form the steps. A complete subunit of the DNA molecule is a base plus backbone-unit.

We will make up compound units for each base—(A + backbone) . . . (C + backbone)—creating something like a vertebra with rib attached. When we link the vertebrae, the ribs will align in parallel steps. Instead of making a double helix, though, we'll concentrate on a single strand of DNA. Each of the bases has a slightly different shape. Although the complementary pairs (AT, GC) are fairly congruent, the face each base presents outward is unique, as unique as a separate letter of the alphabet.

Now we arrange the molecules in a line according to what we want produced. We will make up a backbone with its base-plates facing out in the particular order coding for a particular protein, and the series of letters required to get *one protein* we will call *one gene.*

A gene is nothing more than a region along a DNA chain. It has no obvious physical appearance on the long chain of base plates. A gene is that region which codes for one complete protein.

Genetic code is really considerably simpler than human language. Every "word" is composed of three "letters," so AAT is one word in genetic code, and GGC is another.

The genes are in the nucleus; the proteins are manufactured out in the workshop, the cellular cytoplasm. How do we get the message from one place to another? With the messenger RNA mentioned earlier. Like a wise construction engineer, nature has taken pains to protect the blueprint originals, keeping the DNA always in the nucleus, and sending out photocopies into the hurly-burly of the construction site. A simple solution (and therefore often repeated): the bases stick together complementarily. So why not carry the genetic message in the form of a single complementary chain of nucleotides (nucleic acid units)? Done. The messenger RNA is composed of the same bases, with one exception: The physically similar base uracil replaces thymine of DNA.

Let's say a gene is "turned on." For now, we will understand this highly complex process as nothing more than this: A messenger RNA is assembled complementary to its gene, side by side with it.

When the complete gene is read out, a signal follows that enables the messenger RNA to float free. It slips through the nuclear membrane and floats out into the cytoplasm. There it links up with the cell's workbenches, the ribosomes, referred to earlier as meatballs; like many a meatball they are composed of several ingredients, some known and others unfortunately mysterious. Among the constituents are two different forms of RNA.

The long strand of messenger RNA binds at its head to the ribosome; in fact, one of the codes along the gene region of the DNA was a "ribosome binding site," a configuration of bases particularly attractive to the configurations on the ribosome. Just as a computer punch tape is read out, the RNA physically moves along the ribosome. Enter the final actors in the protein production, a still-different form of RNA called transfer RNA. Transfer RNA joins both worlds: the nucleic acid of DNA/RNA, and the building blocks of protein, amino acids. Each transfer RNA has at its nucleic-acid end the three-letter complement for one three-letter "word" on the messenger. At its protein end it carries the amino acid specified by that "word." It's just as though here at the workbench we had all the parts needed to assemble a protein, and each was tagged with its proper name. On the ribosome workbench, each three-letter word of the messenger RNA is translated via transfer RNA into an amino acid. The amino acids are strung together into a protein chain.

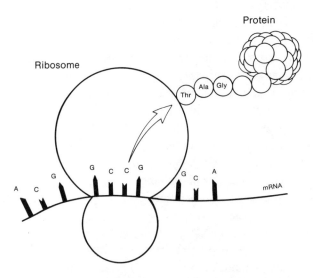

Figure 10. *Close-up of the translation process shown in Figure 7. The genetic code translates three-base "words" of nucleic acids (ACG-GCC-GGC) into amino acid units of protein. The triplets shown here code respectively for the amino acids threonine, alanine, and glycine.*

There are twenty amino acids, and all the thousands of different proteins, structural or enzymatic, of a living organism are simply different combinations and numbers of these twenty amino acids (see Figure 10).

A protein first is simply a chain of amino acids in a particular order, but then this string of beads folds up into a characteristic bunch. Because each amino acid has a different shape and different levels of electrical charge at different places, the protein's final three-dimensional shape will be precisely determined by the order and number of amino acids in its string. That shape is very important to the function of each different protein, whether it is to be a cellular building block or an enzyme. In fact, an enzyme is able to bring about the union of two molecules generally because its shape allows it to serve as a template for the finished product.

All of this takes place under the mediation of vastly more enzymes than I've mentioned, but that is pretty much the whole process: A gene's message is transcribed onto messenger RNA, called transcription because the language remains the same, that of nucleic-acid base units. The messenger RNA travels out to the cytoplasm where, on the ribosomes, it is translated into protein, translated because the language is converted from that of nucleic acids (DNA/RNA) to that of amino acids (protein).

Some of these proteins are wanted in enormous quantity, all the time, so you might find their genes in many copies throughout the DNA complement; more frequently, you will find strong promoters just upstream of the genes, promoters that can bind RNA polymerase tightly and often; and finally you will find enhancers in their neighborhood—the distinction of enhancers being that they are able to exert their influence whether upstream or downstream of the gene whose expression they enhance.

Some of the proteins we want in very small quantity, but to be present all the time; expect to find only a few copies of the gene in the entire genome, but perhaps there will be nothing interfering with their transcription into messenger RNA.

The tricky ones to figure are those proteins that are wanted now in a huge quantity, then not at all, then again in a lesser amount than the first time; these are the proteins whose production is under the strictest and most complex of controls.

If tumor production is the result of unregulated growth and division, then what are the mechanisms of regulation that are lost or damaged? Although the picture is far from complete, the pieces that have emerged at least indicate that the path we're on is the right one. For example, there is the translocation in Burkitt's lymphoma mentioned earlier. We have chromosome number 8, the proper address of thousands of genes, including the oncogene *myc*; now a piece including *myc* is broken off. We have chromosome 14, correct location for thousands of other particular genes, and a piece is broken from it. The two pieces get tacked onto the opposite chromosomes, resulting in a mutant (see Figure 11). That real translocation has been known for years to occur in Burkitt's; as Weinberg noted, it can be seen under an ordinary light microscope. But when Michael Cole and Grace Shen Ong discovered only a few years ago that in the translocation, *myc* wound up directly in front of the promoter for the immunoglobulin gene, there was a wonderful piece of evidence for the importance of gene controls. Immunoglobulin is a blood protein required in huge quantity whenever the body is fighting infection; therefore it would have to be under the control of a powerful promoter. The function of the protein encoded by *myc* is unknown, but wouldn't it be logical that it was a protein involved in growth stimulus, to be expressed very rarely? Burkitt's lymphoma might be the result of the overfrequent expression of *myc*.

But then, it might not. The translocation might be some sort of error that occurs *because* the cell has gone out of whack due to the disease called cancer; it might be the effect of cancer, not the cause. So it rests: Many such chromosomal abnormalities have been discovered in human cancers, several activated oncogenes have been isolated from human tumors, but the precise pathway remains unknown. And even with that pathway fully described, we have reached the level of duplicating only a benign tumor, a lump, a growth; we will have explained how the damaged DNA mistakenly says "Multiply," but not how it gives that final deadly instruction, "Go forth."

But in 1984 in the cancer story, illuminating discoveries would be made concerning these pathways to growth and the genes that con-

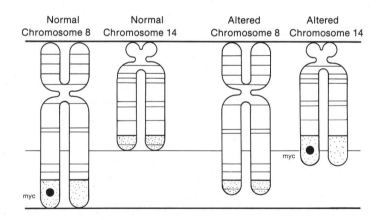

Figure 11. A schematic rendering of the translocation in Burkitt's lymphoma, which can be seen under a light microscope with the chromosome stained to show banding. The arm of chromosome 8, known to contain the normal cellular version of the oncogene myc, *winds up on chromosome 14. Though not mutated,* myc *now is in front of "hot" controls on chromosome 14. Those controls normally regulate antibody production.*

trol them, including discoveries made by one of the scientists I had been relying on to fill me in—Lew Cantley. They are discoveries at a further range, suggesting sweeping answers to the most nagging questions that arise now that oncogenes seem to be proliferating in number: What do oncogenes do? More of that later. But notice that if we speak of a cell proliferating, multiplying out of control, the DNA must be ordering such reproduction and must be reproducing itself. How DNA does replicate itself is one of the marvels of nature, showing how the molecule's shape and function are perfectly entwined.

As a cell divides into two daughter cells, the most important step is to duplicate the DNA complement and split it between the two daughters. DNA's structure is the key to this. The molecule literally unzips, little by little, and with the aid of enzymes, complementary bases floating free in the nucleus are assembled along each unzipping half; in other words, a new whole DNA molecule forms along each half. And the DNA codes, finally, for those enzymes that enable it to reproduce, making this molecule self-reflecting, as bewildering and beguiling as a hall of mirrors. The enzymes make possible chemical reactions that cause assembly of a new DNA molecule, among whose genes are those coding for the enzymes that make possible chemical reactions . . . on and on.

We have here a remarkable theatrical invention: a script that tells how to assemble the actors from available parts, how to energize them, and finally, how each part of each should move and when, to carry out the play from opening curtain to final bow. And in at least the beginning phases of cancer, we seem to be putting on a production of *The Sorcerer's Apprentice*.

Recap: Every cell in your body contains exactly the same DNA (discounting errors). So how does the DNA in a skin cell "know" it should express genes for skin proteins? Meanwhile DNA in cells of the bone marrow expresses genes to build white blood cells but does *not* express epithelial proteins. At the same time, DNA in hair follicle cells "knows" it must express large quantities of the tough protein keratin in a continuous strand, turning the cell into a little wire mill for hair.

You can carry these questions all the way back to that single fertilized egg that once was you, watch it multiply at first just like a bacterium until it consists of about 16 identical cells called a blastocyst. Suddenly different cells begin going three distinctly different ways; some will produce descendants whose eventual descendants will be inner organ cells (endoderm), some will lead to skeletal and other structural cells (mesoderm), and the third group will give ultimate rise to cells of the skin (ectoderm).

* * *

Obviously, this whole process of development and growth occurs using the same set of instructions because different portions are read out. That means that regulation of gene expression is the key to that development, as key as it is to the mis-development of cancer, marking a throwing off of controls and a return to that first, primitive state, when the cell was alone and needed only to grow as quickly as possible.

At Dana–Farber, George Canellos reminded me that the fetus growing in its mother's womb has virtually all the growth-control characteristics of the tumor: It is a foreign cell, yet anchors in the womb and somehow sends signals that prevent its rejection, it invades the mother's blood supply for nourishment, and it grows explosively fast. The fetus lacks only these qualities of cancerous growth: It stays put, barring miscarriage, and it differentiates, week by week, cell group by group and finally cell by cell, into human form; regardless of how many growth controls are not operating, a good many are, and in the closest cooperation.

It seems, looked at up close, that if you could understand this process, you would serendipitously understand cancer; or that if you could understand cancer, reductionistically understand it, you would be a long way toward understanding this fetal development. Now, which is more important? At last, a question we *don't* need to concern ourselves with. The advantage of this fundamental approach of basic science is that if the questions you dedicate yourself to are important enough, solving one problem solves many simultaneously. Isn't that what fundamental means? And doesn't that make perfectly clear Luis Parada's comments on his future when he said it was in developmental biology and gene regulation, not, strictly speaking, in cancer research, but truly related.

Developmental biology indeed is the theme of the Whitehead

Institute, a consistent intellectual focus forged by David Baltimore as the institute's director, Weinberg says. July now, and even as he speaks there is thumping and sliding out in the hall as boxes accumulate up and down the corridors of the Weinberg–Baltimore lab at the cancer center. There are boxes of general laboratory equipment, all scrupulously labeled and coded so they will be delivered to the right rooms at the Whitehead. And of even more vital, if local, importance are each researcher's equipment, chemicals, cultures, notebooks. They are all still out, in use, but in one swoop—speaking of close regulation—they will have to be gathered up, packed, and delivered.

The move will cover a distance of perhaps two hundred yards horizontally, vertically down five floors and up three. But the coordination and the work are the same as if the whole gang were headed for California; only the ride in the moving van is shorter. The ride in the moving van is this short:

> The Whitehead Institute for Biomedical Research began to occupy its handsome new building at the edge of the MIT campus in Cambridge, Massachusetts last week with all the informality of a commune moving day. Graduate students and senior faculty alike were lugging boxes of equipment across the street. At one stage, Dr. Robert A. Weinberg, wearing a yellow and blue striped rugby jersey, was to be seen on the tailboard of a moving van protecting his rubber plant, now 14 years old.
>
>   —item in *Nature*, August 1984

13

Grappling

The foyer of the new Baltimore–Weinberg laboratories is done in burgundy, or it will be; it's now a jumble of half-constructed settees in what will be an attractive anteroom. Down the hall are the secretaries, beyond them Weinberg's office, and as you head for that office the laboratories spread out over the whole of the third floor to your left.

Weinberg has grants on his mind today; they have been on his mind all summer, a real worry over the past six months. Grantsmanship, to many if not most academics, is a vital part of their jobs. It relates to how well they can interest review committees, generally composed of their peers, in the work they are doing and propose to do. But to a scientist running a major laboratory, grants are the very lifeblood of the research operation: no grant, no salary for postdocs or lab technicians, no chemicals, no mice, no nothing; the laboratory would be a dry, impotent hulk, a collection of equipment. It is not unusual for a major university to hire someone based on the number, amount, and quality of grants he or she may bring in, so worry over such matters is hardly trivial; nor is it unusual for a university to grant or withhold tenure from a talented, high-achieving, well-funded scientist because the direction of his or her research is not one the department chooses to follow.

There is a certain black humor in Weinberg's dilemma, he

acknowledges, with such money worries coming in a time of success. "My work always has been well funded, and I've never had to worry about support," he says. "But in the last six months I've been extremely worried, in part because I let my laboratory grow too large, beyond what the grant proposal would support. Ironically, as my work has been reasonably successful I find myself in an economic crisis."

Nevertheless, Weinberg believes that this financial hurdle is a temporary one: "I hope I'll be in a situation several months down the pike where I don't have to worry about it again for a long time. I think it's going to pass. It would not be rational for me to assume I'll have long-term problems with funding." He says he has never been unable to carry out an important project because of lack of funds.

Where does the money come from to support the experiments conducted in all these molecular biology laboratories? By and large from two sources: the National Cancer Institute and other arms of the National Institutes of Health, and the National Science Foundation (NSF). There are literally hundreds of other sources, ranging from large charities like the American Cancer Society to small bequests. However, of some $2 billion annually pumped into cancer research, just about half comes from NCI; other NIH agencies and the NSF provide between 10 and 15 percent, and the remainder comes from nonprofit organizations (also 10 to 15 percent), labor and industry (the same), and state and local governments (about 10 percent).

To get a grant, you first make a lengthy and detailed application; some grant applications cover planned experiments and funds for as long as seven years, and five-year plans are common. The application goes to Washington, where in general a committee of other scientists in your own specialty reviews that application, as you might review one of theirs. (This might seem a conflict but in fact is the cornerstone of what every scientist I spoke to believes is the best scientific enterprise in the world.) That the system functions at all is initially surprising, given the catch-22 that must be overcome from the start.

Put simply and in virtually the same terms by Weinberg, Cantley, Sato, Traktman, and Klotz: There is usually little relationship between what one proposes to do with grant money and what one actually does with it. The reason is simple. According to Cantley, any scientist who knows what he or she is going to be doing in five years is not much of a scientist. In fact, if you're any good at all, you probably don't know what you're going to be doing in six months, let alone five years. Six months is, in fact, less time than it ever takes to have a grant actually funded, with an account number to pay the bills.

What to do? All that you can do. As Weinberg says, what you propose to do in your grant is what you now think you will be doing, what now excites you. In turn, the only thing the peer reviewers can do is to evaluate proposals based on their knowledge of the applicants as scientists. "Have I done good work in the past? Am I reputable?" And finally, they will judge whether, in the view of each, the project is doable. Of course, if the project is as exciting and as doable as the application attests, it is probably being done on a grant already in the bank, a grant that was awarded to do something entirely different. The virtue of the current system, Weinberg points out, is that the reviewers know all that. Neither he nor anyone else interviewed believed that the peer review system needed major improvement. Did cronyism sometimes influence decisions? If a reviewer supported a less-than-outstanding proposal by a current or one-time collaborator (and everyone basically knows everyone else), the other members of the panel would judge him or her accordingly. If by contrast (as is more likely in such competitive science) a reviewer attacked a worthy proposal because it was from a competitor or for a project the panelist had failed at, that would be quickly spotted by other reviewers.

Klotz noted that despite the certainty that no good scientist will adhere to a five-year plan, such concrete proposals allow agencies to monitor changes in direction, which must be accounted for by grantees.

Earlier, when Cantley had talked about his three categories of experiments, he mentioned that some scientists spent their lives generally in category I. A small minority, they are people who may have begun full of excitement about their field, but at some point were stunted by a success—became known for one discovery and clung securely to it. As such a scientist, Cantley said, "You'll get funding. You'll do the work. In fact, you'll do exactly the experiments you propose. There are a fair number of people out there who really do not break new ground and don't care to. They always know what they'll be doing five years from now. You do have to wonder if they ever wind up in the governmental bureaucracy, deciding whether other scientists ought to be funded or not."

Weinberg, like any major laboratory head, also has many different grants he is administering at any given moment, all of different amounts, many operating under different guidelines, and most neither beginning nor ending at the same time. To make sure that everyone gets paid and the lab's checks don't bounce requires no end of juggling, and there are few things scientists find more annoying than a notification from the government that funds that were used to pay, say, a technician's salary were misused, because they were granted to pay something else. Cantley observed, "I'm administering two grants right now. I write all my checks on one of them. When it runs out, I'll start writing checks on the other one."

Weinberg says of the accounting: "It's all a charade. In the end I get grants from four or five different sources, and each one allegedly is hooked to one project, but it's all ridiculous because the projects shift from month to month and I have no idea which money is used for what. But in the end it all has to be rationalized in terms of a certain one."

A few months later Paula Traktman would go through the first throes of being a "principal investigator": setting up her own laboratory at Cornell University Medical College. "One month you're a postdoc, worrying about your own experiments, your own work. And the next month you're staring at an empty laboratory. I have an equipment grant, and all I've done is run around checking prices, to make sure I can buy the equipment for the amount of the grant." It is what Huki Land looks forward to next year, with a natural mix of eagerness and apprehension. Still later in the summer I would spend time with Mike Kriegler, who had just set up his own laboratory at Philadelphia's Fox Chase cancer institute after completing a postdoc at Berkeley.

His experience: "That's a tough and scary time, going out on your own. And it changes some people. You can talk to people in a big lab, and they all sound very daring and experimental, but in a year they're kind of looking over the edge. They're not in somebody else's lab anymore, the symbiosis isn't there; they're supposed to put it together. Some people at that point just decide to play it safe."

And there are the horror stories. While dining at the Cantleys, Lynn Klotz related the saga of a young scientist he knew who had been an assistant professor at Harvard and was interested in slime molds. These are very primitive multicelled organisms that are differentiated into only a few types of tissue. Scientists are forever seeking model systems. Since slime molds are primitive, they offer a simple system to study differentiation stripped away from the jungle of genetic apparatus involved in differentiation of higher animals. However, slime molds fell out of favor as experimental systems because development now could be studied at a higher level. So the young scientist found himself out of a job—not for failing, but because his experimental system had gone out of fashion.

What next? That certainly is a prospect many other people in many other fields have faced, and more than once. But Klotz notes: "The difference here is that you have someone in whom society has invested a great deal of money, in training that goes on, by the doctoral level, for many, many years. And suddenly that's all brought to a halt. Maybe not a permanent one, but the threat to him at this juncture is very serious. Most people that highly trained in other fields don't face that kind of dead end."

Still, Weinberg and many others believe that overall funding in their own subspecialty has not been too low—perhaps a surprising admission. Weinberg noted how explosively the field of oncogene research had grown during the 1980s. While conceding that the number in the field "is certainly larger than the number of those who are productive," he added, "it's one of the glories of American science that the system is so flexible people can leap fields as something new and exciting opens up," he said. "And given what's happened in oncogenes, I think it's good that so many people are interested. That tends to confirm that this is an important and legitimate field of inquiry." But in terms of funding: "I think it's quite adequately funded, and I'm not at all convinced that increasing the funds would improve the quality of the work. Sometimes, in fact, the opposite is the effect. When there's a lot of money floating around, people start proposing experiments without really thinking of whether they're necessary. When money's tight, that forces you to sit down and whittle away till you come up with what's really important, and that can make the field move faster."

Such optimism was hardly universal in cancer research in 1984. As summer drew to a close there were ominous reports of major investigators who had scored very high with their review committees being cut off without grants. Sharp cutbacks in funding, some intended by Congress, others initiated by the Office of Management and the Budget, were to leave many in both basic and clinical sciences dangling without funds.

Weinberg noted that the speed with which investigators have migrated into oncogenes is a just climax for the past years of cancer research. "For two decades much of basic biology has been justified on the basis of its importance to cancer research. It was all a ploy to get money, a quite necessary ploy. And in retrospect, it worked: All these areas of [such as viral models] proved keys to oncogenesis."

Making a field move fast is of course what people like Weinberg are interested in, and moving it, whenever possible, within the confines of their own laboratories. There are exigencies involved here that also help explain the difficulty of literal accounting for grants. Graduate students, for example, are not around for more than a few years. "It takes six to twelve months for them to get a project moving, and if it doesn't show promise by then we usually get them to rethink what they're doing, because they're usually under great pressure to do something in two to three years time, and I don't want them to leave empty-handed," says Weinberg.

It is important for the new "doctor" to have his or her name on publications, an even more important requirement by the end of the postdoctoral fellowship nearly all scientists carry out. The particular journal by which the publication is accepted is important; in any given field there are only a handful considered at the top, a second ranking, and finally journals that scientists know will, in the words of Cantley, "publish almost anything."

How does it evolve that an experiment or a series of experiments become a paper?

"There's a poorly defined set of criteria as to what constitutes a body of work," Weinberg said. "It's dependent on the discipline and the subdiscipline. But there's a point where one has a natural feeling that the amount of data has developed so one can tell a nice story about a given thing, that one has a series of results which present some coherent, logical flow, which are not an isolated bit of information but a corpus."

Still, Weinberg says that topicality plays a key role. "On occasion, I'll say to somebody, okay, let's start writing it up. I might even ask them to start writing it up before they finish it as a goad to doing the writing and as a goad to thinking through the ramifications of their experimental work."

The order of the names on the article is of great importance. Weinberg had said earlier that each of the people in his laboratory was "a prime investigator in his or her own project." Weinberg himself holds the title of principal investigator, a formal term indicating that he is the person responsible for the grant money, the one running the lab.

"The people doing the work, the ones most involved, should be first," said Weinberg. "I invariably am last, unless there's collaboration with another laboratory, which complicates the order." Weinberg assigns the writing to that prime investigator, in general, but usually rewrites the result, becoming an editor. "I'll sit and justify each of my revisions. It might be the clarity of the logic, the logical flow of ideas, or the clear integration of the whole flow of ideas. For many this represents their first experience of putting out a scientific paper, and I think it is a useful one. I like to think our papers are well written and clear. I impress upon people that a poorly written paper is a sign of a poorly thinking mind." But he adds, "There are a lot of good scientists who just are not able to express themselves very well, either because they are inarticulate or because they don't have much of a pedagogical sense of what other people will or won't understand."

Determining which journal to shoot for: "I'll suggest one, but I tell them that it's their paper. Here are the considerations: How rapidly will they publish? How long is the paper? Which journal gives the best reproduction of figures? Which journals have reasonable referees and which are sticklers for what we might consider unreasonable, minute details?" And finally, of course, "What's the audience? —and is it the right one for this paper?"

Publication is linked to grantsmanship in two ways. First, granting agencies look to articles for evidence that the grant money has been effective. Second, publications show the quality and direction of an investigator's work. But the real importance of publication has more to do with a scientist's professional standing. Most scientists are very sensitive to the judgment of their peers, a judgment formed to a large extent by the work published in quality journals.

By the end of their time with him, Weinberg begins to try to gain his scientists public exposure, through meetings as well as publications. Scientific meetings are yet another aspect of the critical mass of brainpower, concentrated on a single problem or related problems, that lies at the core of modern science.

But not all his alumni will go into academic science. Many will head into the burgeoning—and well-paying—industries involved in genetic engineering and related fields of biotechnology. Cambridge is home to more of these corporations than any other area except San Francisco, not surprising since both areas are so deeply involved in the most advanced biological research. The coming of these industries and their effect on "pure research" conducted in universities has gotten mixed reviews from scientists, but there is one aspect of their growth that is positive from this vantage point: They provide jobs.

Weinberg says, "With our field growing so explosively, if I were to put out only two graduate students a year from my laboratory, since there is only one of me, you can see we've got exponential growth. There obviously are not enough university laboratories in the country for all these people to find places."

Looking at the grant process in any given year offers a good idea of how scientists have adjusted to their system. Look at the process over a period of years and we get a moving picture of a wrestling match: Funds are now loose, now tight, inflation intensifies, subsides. To each change in forces the scientist must respond to keep the lab operating, the experiments under way, the postdocs in fellowships. Looking down a corridor of more than a dozen years, we can now see the effects of these funding changes—changes that have been severe in recent years.

Action–reaction: By 1983, federal budget cutbacks were already having major effects on how scientists proceeded with grant applications. I begin with 1983 because the final figures are available and the current effects were by then all beginning to be felt, but it was, in Cantley's words, "the last good year."

Cantley reviews general medical grants in physical biochemistry, serving on review committees for direct-NIH rather than NCI grants. By 1985—the review year for grants to be funded in 1986—only 15 percent of the grants approved by Cantley's NIH peer review committee and the overseeing government councils were actually being funded. At the NCI, officially, 35 percent of approved grants were being funded.

However, Jerry Boyd, who publishes the respected insider-newsletter *The Cancer Letter*, says the figure is actually more like 25 percent. For fiscal 1986, congress approved funding 6,500 "new or competing renewal" grants, the number considered most significant in judging the state of cancer research funding. But the office of Management and the Budget wanted that number cut to 5,000. Because of laws restricting the ability of the executive branch to withhold Congressionally approved money, OMB could not directly stop the awarding of the funds. What OMB did was to insist that some single-year grants be considered multi-year. The effect was precisely the same as cutting the total to 5,000. (Recently, a compromise was struck for 6,000.)

Generally, this is the timetable for the grant process throughout the NIH: If in February a grant proposal is submitted, the appropriate peer committee will review it in June. Sometime in the fall it will be approved for funding or not. If approved, it will be funded the following January or February—a turnaround of about one year.

Consider the immediate consequences of a funding percentage as small as 15 to 25 percent. First, review committees become tougher, pick proposals apart routinely, send many more back with criticisms than ordinarily. "If that happens," says Cantley. "you rewrite the proposal and send it back. Everyone does. Naturally, you'll make at least some alteration in the second proposal." If it comes back again, "you'll write it a third time, with another change, taking the criticisms into account again."

Result: Researchers are spending drastically more time writing grants, less time doing research. Grant review committees are reviewing far more grants, but giving out less money. In other words, there are fewer research dollars, and each research dollar buys less, so the reduction in research moves exponentially downward. The plunge tapers off only when money has been tight for so long that researchers leave the field. As Weinberg says of his own departing postdocs, some young researchers must do so; but Cantley notes that scientists now in their early to mid-forties, who have been doing research for fifteen years, cannot usually afford to do so, and it is generally counterproductive to the field when they do.

When grant applications are reviewed, they are scored by the peer committees on a point system from 100 high to 500 low. According to Vicki Sato, in the heyday of cancer funding in the early 1970s a proposal with a score of 250 might be funded. In recent years one could expect funding with anything lower than a 170 or 180. By 1984, however, scientists with scores above 140 were worried. Paula Traktman, in her first year as a "lab boss," was funded but a friend who scored 158 was not. A year later, in grants reviewed for the 1986 fiscal year, the passing score had dropped to 145 in some cases.

Consider these funding figures published by the NCI's parent National Institutes of Health:

In 1972 the NCI "obligations" for all projects totaled $378.6 million, but they rose quickly in 1973 to $431.2 million and in 1974 to $581 million. The steep climb continued to a peak of just under $1 billion in 1980, dropping back somewhat to $986.8 million by 1983.

But those are "current dollars," unadjusted for the runaway inflation of the 1970s. When the NIH figured the same obligations in so-called "constant" 1972 dollars, the NCI obligation that began at $378.6 million then rose to $411.6 million and $521.4 million for 1974—still large increases. But it peaked at $573.7 million in 1976, the worst inflation year, then began dropping. By 1983, "the good year," NCI funding in inflation-adjusted dollars had fallen to $437 million, not a lot more than the 1972 figure.

How much was being bought for this money? In 1973, the first year the NIH shows figures for calculating award percentages, the NCI funded 484 grants, 54 percent of those approved by the peer review committees and overseeing councils. By 1983, 886 grants were awarded—nearly double the initial number—but they represented only 33.9 percent of the number approved, a drop of nearly 20 percent. Further, grant dollar amounts had dropped considerably, and the combination lends credence to Cantley's assertion that a scientist who formerly would have run his or her lab on one or two large grants, written and reviewed once, is now scrambling to collect larger numbers of smaller grants, using more time in grantsmanship and proportionally less in research. Similarly, more review panels have to review that larger number of grants.

Further, in 1973, the NCI approval rate of 54 percent was far above the NIH average of 38.9 percent. By 1983 it was second lowest: The 33.9 percent approval rate of NCI compares with a 37.2 percent NIH average by then.

Throughout the NIH, in 1972 the average grant size was $57,600. In constant dollars, by 1983 the average had dropped to $54,800. This proliferation of increasingly smaller grants has been accompanied by yet another critical change: Indirect costs, or overhead, have shot up. The terms refer to a controversial and very "soft" number that is taken out of grants, after they've been awarded, by universities and research institutes, as their entitlement. The grantee must pay a percentage back to the university to cover the cost of the laboratory space, services, utilities, and so forth. Overhead is really a charge assessed to the granting organization. The idea is that if, say, the NCI gets a research project carried out at Harvard or MIT or Cold Spring Harbor, it is getting the use of everything those major institutions have to offer in facilities and support. The NIH, unlike the National Science Foundation, includes this overhead charge in the grant total, where it is not visible. Over the years, the percentages of grants going to overhead have risen considerably and have even come to include reimbursement for large portions of the researcher's own salary—formerly paid entirely by the university or institute.

Here's how the overhead percentages changed from 1973 to 1983 among the three major types of organizations involved in cancer research.

Universities:	from 23.1 percent to 30.3 percent
Research institutes:	from 25.8 percent to 33.6 percent
Hospitals:	from 18.5 percent to 24.6 percent

In other words, if a researcher got a substantially larger grant in 1983 than ten years previously, once the sum was converted to constant dollars and the larger percentage of overhead was deducted, the real amount might have fallen considerably. But that's just an average for all grants. For a particular grant, from which a salary reimbursement is to be deducted, the university might demand that the grant cover 60 percent of the researcher's annual salary. Say an M.D. researcher's salary, including all fringe benefits, was $140,000— a not-unrealistic figure—the university might ask for his or her grants to cover $70,000.

That's not saying that this money handed over to a university is squandered or devoted to nonresearch ends, but the organization is not as accountable for it as the researcher would be. On most university campuses with a strong research component a controversy erupts periodically over whether the administrator in charge of overhead is using the money as a "slush fund" to bolster undergraduate education or for another use unrelated to research. I've never known one of those controversies to be resolved with the revelation of hard figures—and that's what I mean by "accountable."

Considering all this, the draw by the NCI of top researchers is easy to understand. "Intramural" NCI scientists do not have to apply for grants. Their work is funded, perhaps not as extensively as they would wish, but in the words of several, support is "more or less guaranteed" by virtue of their being hired on. They must withstand more political pressure concerning what they investigate; that is the tradeoff. But they do not face the prospect of finding that a grant score that put them near the top of the heap was not close enough to the top, that they must now grapple for a new handhold.

PART III

LIGHTS AND TUNNELS

14

Night

Anonymity: an American city at nightfall, the only natural light a watermelon-red slash in the west, in counterpoint to all that is not natural. The buildings' aluminum and glass, setting forth their own starfields, could be anywhere in the country. A Greyhound bus, conical reading light defining an inner world at least as anonymous. The bus plunges now out of that world, into a green tunnel, the world inside a neon tube; then after a hundred yards out into the night. Checkerboard lights that say nothing of the shapes that project them; no form emerging out of darkness, just lights and dark and shapes made strange by random interplay. Into another tunnel, out; plunging, re-emerging, the end of each the signal for the other to begin.

The rider puts on the headset and turns the tape recorder on, begins transcribing. The first thing the doctor, who is a medical oncologist, says is that anonymity is required here. And the story has to be checked, but it will check. And here, in sum, is what was said; the whole of it comes later.

The most prestigious and far-reaching breast cancer studies in the United States have been carried out under the direction of Dr. Bernard Fisher, head of the National Surgical Adjuvant Breast Project (NSABP) in Pittsburgh. Fisher has a reputation both as a brilliantly perceptive scientist and a man of unquestionable integrity, one who would interpret the data as cleanly as they could be interpreted, whether the knife edge fell for or against him. It was Fisher's group that had developed, carefully and painstakingly, the set of treatment protocols followed for breast cancer throughout the United States. Beginning with certain suppositions based on their concept of the biology of breast cancer, they had posited a combination of surgery (radical or total mastectomy, lumpectomy), particular chemotherapy combinations, and radiation to be administered for a woman in a given classification. There are many classifications; and cancer specialists around the world are constantly seeing if those need adjustment: What is the effect of age on the severity of a given type of breast tumor? What particular age groups lend themselves to which chemotherapy regimens? But all such protocols are based on suppositions; they had to be tested.

Fisher's group began studies nearly twenty years ago to determine whether the Halsted radical mastectomy was as good a treatment for breast cancer as less severe operations. Now, in late summer 1984, physicians and clinical researchers around the country have already been waiting for months for the results of the most important study the NSABP has ever done, a series of conclusions based on twenty years of data on millions of American women. Never before has such a thorough and scientifically respectable survey been available on which to base treatment decisions.

In a meeting room in Palm Springs in the winter of 1984, Fisher had suddenly ordered the doors closed, and with a voice of authority told those assembled that they must not spread what they were about to hear beyond the doors. He was about to report the findings on one of the major protocols of his co-investigators, the other members of the NSABP from around the country; for reasons that would soon be apparent, he was concerned not that they might spread the results by word of mouth, but that they might appear in some publication prematurely.

The results of this massive study, Fisher announced, showed that across the board there appeared to be no difference in survival rates for women who had had simple mastectomies versus those who had had mere lumpectomies. Dead silence. Fisher was proving twenty years of his own work, and the hard results matched those inferred from his understanding of the biology of cancer, of how it spread. Why the secrecy? Because across the United States in thousands of hospitals, the way doctors treated their patients might change as a result. Ironically, most doctors had already begun moving to less radical forms of breast-cancer treatment, not a few of them because they believed that Fisher's biology was right.

Based largely on Fisher's preliminary work, few Halsted radical mastectomies were performed any longer. These were the most-disfiguring operations in which not only breast tissue but also underlying musculature was removed. But the indications of protocol BO6, which Fisher was now reporting, went beyond that: simple mastectomy, the removal of all breast tissue, did not appear to improve survival over mere lumpectomies with and without radiation treatment.

This study had been federally funded, by the NCI, and there could be no erroneous, inflammatory leaks that would distort the results. Further, the only proper place for these findings to come to light was in one of the world's most credible and powerful medical journals: the *New England Journal of Medicine*.

The *New England Journal of Medicine* operates under its own stiff protocol, known as the Inglefinger Rule after the former editor who proclaimed it: Any paper proposed for publication in the journal whose results are broached in any other publication will not be accepted for publication in the journal. Fisher did not mention the Inglefinger rule, nor did he need to. This landmark study with all the conclusions to be drawn from it had only one proper showcase, one medium where its results would be trusted and seen in their proper light, and nothing was going to risk that publication.

And here is why the doctor repeated the story, the tale transcribed from its tape on a night bus ride: Now it was six months later, and still the Journal *had not published the study, nor had it been sent back to permit submission elsewhere. Not even the most powerful cancer physicians and bureaucrats in the country had been able to dislodge it, and frustration continued to build through ensuing months as this powerful force—the NSABP studies—was hung up in the scientific review process, yet hung up long beyond the reasonable time for peers and editors to review it. Another eight frustrating months would pass before publication—a total of more than a year between one frame of reference and the next for oncologists around the United States. When the studies finally emerged after a delay of*

14 months, the only explanation from the journal was that intensive review had been needed, and from Fisher came an exasperated acceptance.

Out of the city now, the countryside, pure black, vanishes, leaving the dimly lit bus its own little world of readers and snorers, chatterers, cryers, smokers, headset listeners.

15

Feedback

An early briskness has fallen over New England, a welcome end to a hot, rainy summer. Back in the laboratory area of the newly occupied Whitehead, the only surprise is that among all the gleaming new equipment, the more things change, the more they stay the same. The same graffiti greet the eyes, the same blue binders lie in their deceptive apparent disorder. On the wall an ever-crazed "Doctor Land" finds that rats are the cause of cancer, and on the benches all around the same tubes are drying on upturned plastic fingers; the 1966 Orioles remain on the front page of the *Baltimore Sun*, immortalized. Most important, the same people are still bouncing ideas off one another, the chatter running fast and free up and down the corridors, in and out of laboratory doors.

It has been two years now since Huki Land arrived in Weinberg's lab, more than a year since he found that *myc* plus *ras* would accomplish the deadly magic that no single oncogene had—complete transformation of a normal cell. On the Fourth of July he had been looking for new oncogene pairs to accomplish the same feat, and now as summer wound into fall he had new success. But why the excitement over yet another powerful oncogene pair? Discovering the potency of *myc* and *ras* together, of course, overcame the serious challenge to Weinberg's original transfaction experiments: that only the already somewhat decontrolled NIH3t3 cells would lose all control and proliferate under the action of an oncogene. But what was the interest in further combinations?

I found part of the answer as I sat at Parada's bench, reading an article by Michael Bishop and trying to piece together the pathway science has taken to this place in the oncogene story. We come now, in roughly the order molecular biologists themselves did, to the next major quest in the search for the molecular basis of cancer, the search for what oncogenes do. By this time about two dozen onco-genes had been located—not counting the one Alan Schechter was at this moment describing down the hall here, an oncogene he and Weinberg would name *neu* and which Weinberg would introduce at *Nature's* cancer conference in Boston the next month.

But *neu* or not, the discovery of additional oncogenes is not the major aim of Weinberg or the other leading labs in cancer research, and understanding the aim helps show the importance of Land's work.

Bishop's article is entitled "Oncogenes Come of Age"—appropriate to the "father of the oncogene." Like Weinberg, Bishop is a clear and lucid writer, his style elegant, at once heavy on latinate words and powerfully descriptive: "It seems likely that the growth and di-vision of cells are regulated by an interdigitating network spanning from the surface of the cell to the heart of the nucleus."

A wonderful entry point for this new labyrinth, the activity of oncogenic proteins. Interlace the splayed fingers of two hands, then send a signal, a touch, moving in a wave from one finger to the next; watch the rolling ball at the Science Museum smack into a row of standing balls, itself stopping, transferring its energy and sending the last ball ripping off. Interdigitating networks, analogous to the network of messengers spanning from the cell surface to the depths of the nucleus, where genes lie silent until triggered by the proper message, and then are expressed. Hormones, steroids, and other vital regulatory proteins called growth factors all work by influencing these intracellular messenger proteins, this interdigitating network (Figure 12).

These regulators are not produced by the cells they influence. Some, like hormones, are produced in parts of the body very distant from the cell system they regulate. All operate in much the same

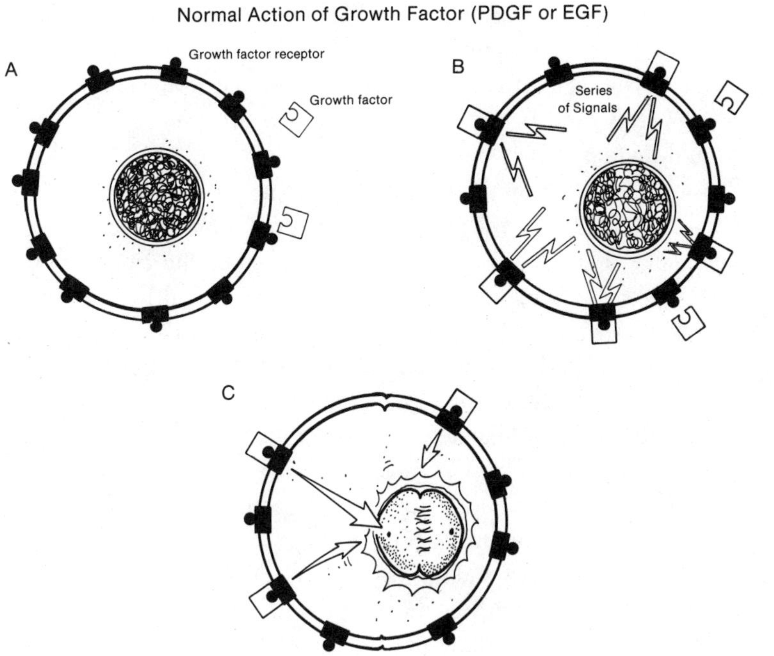

Normal Action of Growth Factor (PDGF or EGF)

Figure 12. *Growth factors induce cells to multiply, but are never produced by the cells they regulate. Streaming out of the blood, these proteins latch onto cell-surface receptors, causing many series of signals to be sent within the cell. Final steps in the series cause DNA to multiply and make proteins for daughter cells.*

manner: The regulator molecule has a receptor in the cell's outer surface, like a socket it plugs into. The receptor molecules are fascinating structures. Their "head ends" face outward on the cell membrane and their "tail ends" point inward, sometimes extending all the way through the membrane so the tail ends are part of the inner-cellular environment.

Watch: A regulatory protein streams out of the blood and plugs into the receptor head; this alters the shape or electrical-charge balance of the receptor. The receptor's tail end now becomes activated; that might mean it carries out an enzyme activity inside the cell, or it might latch onto yet another inner-cellular protein, which "interdigitates" with yet another. These messenger pathways can be long or short, the messages sent at lightning speed or slowly. But in the case of the regulatory growth factors the final result is always the same: Within the nucleus, genes are turned on, causing the cell to grow and divide.

Perhaps the most fascinating aspect of such a process is that it's possible nothing but information is conveyed from outside the cell to the genes. The growth factors may never enter the cell; they pass their chemical message in through the receptor, and although it's not known whether they get past the membrane or not, there appears no reason for them to do so in order to carry out their work, which is to stimulate that interdigitating chain of events.

Writes Bishop: "If that network were touched at any point by an adverse influence and thrown out of balance, neoplastic growth might ensue." Of course this is the key to our interest in this kind of signaling process: It seems quite possible that neoplastic, or tumorous, growth results from just such a loss of balance.

That focuses our attention on the growth factors and their receptors first, then on the interdigitating network within, a vital group of molecules Lew Cantley is studying, called second messengers because they mediate between the external regulatory proteins and the genes that must be activated for growth. Network, of course, implies two or more, in cooperation, and that leads toward Land's objective.

When we ask what oncogenes do, there is an obvious complementary question: What do the *normal* versions of the cellular oncogenes do? Knowing this might lead us to what goes wrong in neoplastic growth, and Bishop now turns his attention here. Two growth factors have been studied closely and have yielded startling insights into the process of growth control. They are epidermal growth factor (EGF) and platelet-derived growth factor (PDGF).

EGF is activated when flesh is pierced or abraded. It signals epidermal cells to reproduce, to heal the wound. PDGF is produced by blood platelets as part of the complex process of blood coagulation and tissue repair. So it is easy to understand the excitement that ensued when Michael Waterfield of Cambridge University discovered that the oncogene *erbB* was quite similar, or homologous, to the gene that codes for the EGF *receptor*.

The *erbB* and normal EGF receptor genes are not identical. The oncogene-encoded receptor is truncated, incomplete. Although the effect of that is not known, researchers believe that the damaged receptor may always have its tail end activated, passing to the rest of the network the message that EGF is present when it is not, telling the cell to grow and divide when it should not.

Shortly after Waterfield's discovery, a team at the NCI led by Stuart Aaronson worked out the sequences of the *sis* oncogene of simian sarcoma virus. At the same time, a group including Harry Antoniades of the Harvard School of Public Health and Michael Hunkapillar of Cal Tech reported the sequence of the gene coding for PDGF. Suddenly from the University of California at San Diego came word that *sis* was homologous to PDGF—that is, the *sis* protein was a variation of the growth factor itself rather than the receptor.

The discovery was yet another great expression of the household god Serendipity. Russell Doolittle, chairman of the chemistry department at USCD, keeps a collection of protein sequences on his home computer, and when he fed in the sequence for PDGF he noticed it was very much like the one he had recently entered for the *sis* oncogene.

In this case scientists speculate that the damaged gene *sis* might be turned on in a cell that is supposed to *receive* the growth factor message, not send it. Such a cell would be self-stimulating, sending out growth messages and then responding to them. Or the PDGF might be expressed by the oncogene in the right cells but at inappropriate times, even continuously (see Figure 13 and Figure 14).

Further, in the cases of both PDGF and EGF-receptor, the damaged genetic message would be passed on to daughter cells as chromosomes reproduced, just the kind of escalation of growth signals we imagine occurring in the eruption of a tumor, a closed loop that might form, like the continuing magnification of static in feedback between microphone and speaker.

So the hunt narrows. We may already have seen cancer's first step but don't know it, can't know it, reductionistically, until the steps are linked into a solid causal chain. And that is the significance of Huki Land's continuing search.

*   *   *

"We're just writing it up," Land says. "*Myb* can also complement with *ras*, and *n-myc* has been found by the Bishop group to complement *ras*. All these are able to immortalize cells."

The long strings of awkward names aside, these are oncogenes whose proteins might cooperate, figuratively interdigitating, to form a pathway to oncogenesis. It's interesting that they all complement with *ras*. Has anything been found that is itself *ras*-like?

"*Src* is more *ras*-like," Land said. *Src*, the first-found oncogene, of Peyton Rous's first-found sarcoma virus.

Michael Wigler has questioned to me the certainty of this "two-gene hypothesis" of Land and Parada. "You put in one oncogene and you shake the cell up," he said. "Put in two and you shake it a hell of a lot. I'm not convinced you have more than that there. And then

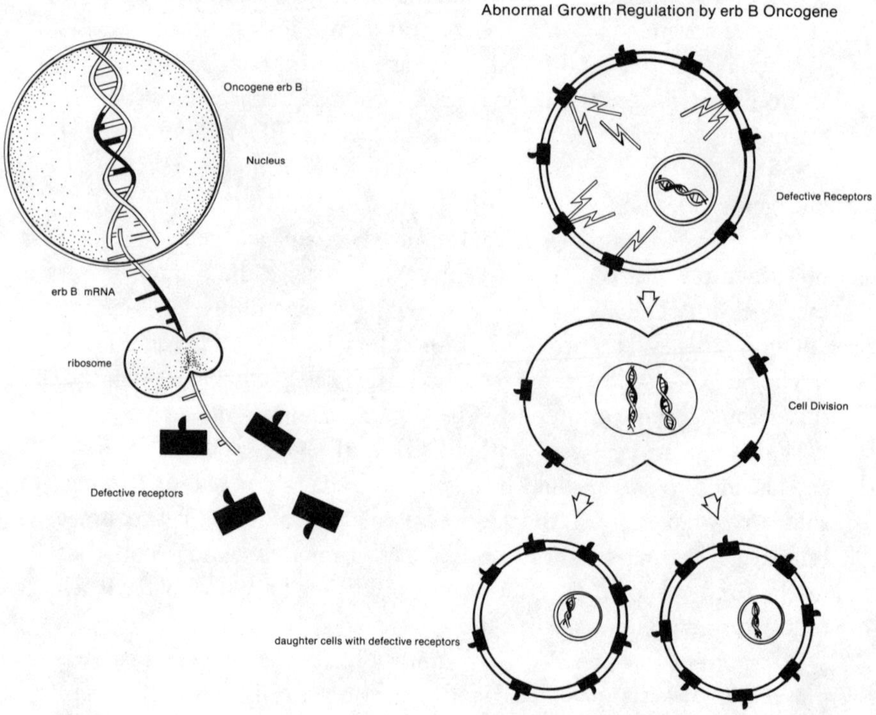

Figure 13. The oncogene erbB codes for a broken receptor for epidermal growth factor (EGF). It may be that this receptor constantly signals the presence of EGF even when none is present, so the cell grows and multiplies constantly at "emergency" speed.

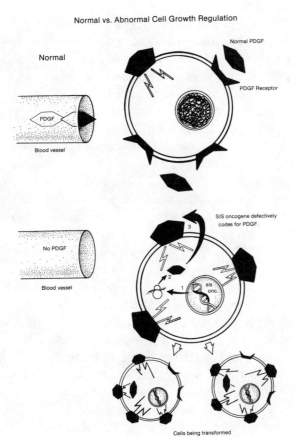

Figure 14. *The sis oncogene was recently found to code for platelet-derived growth factor (PDGF). Scientists speculate that the oncogene may be activated in cells that are supposed to receive PDGF out of the bloodstream, not produce it. Such cells would be self-stimulating and would give rise to daughter cells similarly able to grow and multiply without an external supply of growth factors.*

you take this idea that step one immortalizes and step two transforms."

But doesn't that gibe with a lot of independent evidence concerning the multistep nature of cancer?

"Sure," he said. "But whenever I hear people talking about im-
mortalization I tend to think they don't really know what they mean.
I don't know what that means." Wigler, of course, is expert in mammalian cell lines, the kind to which the term immortalize would apply
if it applies anywhere. And Land himself has pointed out that even
with *myc* and *ras*, the most potent combination yet discovered, all cells
in a culture were not transformed. That suggested to him that a
third, even a fourth oncogene might be at work in those cells that
were transformed.

However, Weinberg fully believes there is more than coincidence
in these cooperations between oncogene pairs, and he believes this
is now proved beyond any mere feeling of certainty. "You find
in vivo tumors with two oncogenes in them, and that's one reason
we believe we're repeating an *in vivo* process. In fact, we've just
found another Burkitt's lymphoma with a *ras* and a *myc*."

But there's more to his certainty. There is also evidence that *ras*
and *myc* exert qualitatively different effects on cells, and the implications of those differences make Weinberg very enthusiastic. "*Ras*
changes cell shape and gives anchorage independence, and it induces
the cells to secrete growth factors"—the first step in the messenger
network. "*Myc* immortalizes cells and causes cells to be more sensitive to these exogenous growth factors." And here again the implications are exciting: One oncogene causes growth factor secretion,
another makes cells more sensitive to those factors.

It is not this experimental complementarity alone that excites
Weinberg and the many other scientists who see cancer as he does,
it is the fact that this fits into a direct pathway, into a reductionist
explanation of oncogenesis: Step 1, *ras* oncogene is mutated . . .
Step n, *myc* oncogene is mutated . . . Step z, when the last, still
mysterious gene in the pathway turns on, the proliferating tumor
acquires all the characteristics needed to metastasize. The secret of
the last step, Weinberg now believes, is being unraveled in his own
laboratory, by Shelly Bernstein. But by "last step" the reductionist
doesn't necessarily mean this temporally final step, but whatever

will be the last piece found. No one knows whether that will turn out to be the key to the metastasis gene or to one of the intermediary steps. And discoveries concerning these intermediaries are what Weinberg had earlier referred to as "largely the work of others"— discoveries about the second messengers, about tongue-twisting phosphatidylinositol and its cousins that provided what one investigator called "seductive evidence" of a completed pathway to the portal of metastasis.

The idea that cancer is a multistep, indeed two-step process owes to work done by Peyton Rous and others in the late 1940s. The question they were trying to answer was: Why was there virtually always a latency period between carcinogen action and the development of tumors? Even people irradiated early in the days of x-ray experiments, when radiation hazards were not known, did not develop tumors immediately.

To compress what was really nearly a half-century of work by many people, experimenters ultimately found that if they applied coal tar to mouse skin, no tumors developed; but if they added croton oil, an irritant, tumors did develop.

The coal tar was acting as an initiator of tumorigenesis, and that initiation turned out to be irreversible; long delays in applying the follow-up carcinogen still resulted in tumors. The croton oil was termed a promoter: a needed second step to push cells over into tumorous growth. Promoters alone would not cause tumors. When experimenters stopped applying promoters, the tumors would stop growing. So promotion was reversible, initiation was not. And this model of cancer development fit with epidemiological findings; people exposed to any number of carcinogens often do not show the effects for many years—until, perhaps, that necessary second (or further?) step is taken.

Croton oil turned out to contain one of the most powerful agents in the cancer pathway, a member of a class of chemicals called phorbol esters. These would prove most interesting—first, because they would turn out *not* to be mutagens; and second, because they would suggest how a large missing piece of the picture of how tumors grow might fall neatly into place, a piece that Cantley would soon explain.

Most carcinogens are mutagens. They combine with the DNA molecule in some way that interferes with its function. However, most of them are initiators in the cancer pathway, not promoters. Like the coal tar rubbed on a mouse's skin, they will cause tumorous growth, but that growth will stop when the initiator is removed. Again, most of the substances we call carcinogens are initiators, e.g., radiation, dioxin, PCBs, polyvinylchloride. The promoters seem, if anything, at least as important in the cancer process. That's where phorbol esters (and substances like tar and asbestos as well) come in. They are not mutagens; they never even enter the cell's nucleus where its DNA resides. Yet they are a class of extremely potent promoters that will rapidly cause cancer in nearly any animal already initiated.

Initiate, promote: the two-step. And how neatly that model fit Land and Parada's discoveries of cooperation between *myc* and *ras*, *myb* and *ras*, and *n-myc* and *ras*, and how *src* behaved like *ras*.

Hard at work searching for the gene or genes that might cause metastasis, Shelly Bernstein finds himself delighted with the atmosphere and equipment in the new laboratories. He is working on the mouse model. From the time of Peyton Rous and the first oncogenic viruses, mice have been used to test the effects of carcinogens and combinations of carcinogens. Because they are mammals, their immune systems are much like our own. In the Whitehead's well-equipped animal lab Bernstein has a separate room with a colony of between 100 and 150 mice. And now he is working not on nude mice but on ordinary "immune competent" white mice of a strain called NFS.

Already, "I had been able to inject human metastases in nude mice and get metastatic growth in them," Bernstein said later. "But I was concerned. They are immune-incompetent; there might be too many reasons for the metastases." The nude mice, after all, were bred to have no defenses against tumors and other illnesses, making them good laboratory subjects—too good. Indeed, a laboratory animal, like an established cell line, could be an artifact; it could produce artifactual results and wrong conclusions.

So far he had had no luck inducing metastases in normal mice. He was following the serial transfection procedure Land and Parada had used, which had been performed in Weinberg's lab for several years by now. He took DNA from human metastatic tumors, broke it into pieces of about 30,000 base pairs each by shearing—squeezing it through a narrow pipette to snap the giant molecule's bonds. He grew cultures of NIH3t3 cells containing the gene bits—some containing transforming genes but, perhaps, others containing genes for metastasis—and injected the grown cultures into the mice. No metastases.

Another of Cantley's category III experiments: The negative answers told you nothing. Lack of metastasis might mean that some significant event was not caused by gene action, as many scientists and doctors believe. Or it might mean that the immune system of the mice were rejecting the protein products expressed by the human genes. The strain of mice Bernstein was now using are genetically the closest to the NIH3t3 strain. He chose them for that reason, figuring the odds on nonrejection were best.

Friday afternoon is greeted in most biology laboratories by the appearance of a tub of ice in some convenient niche, soon followed by bottles and cans of beer and ale. Here in the Whitehead, still awaiting its finishing touches, the niche is the entrance hall, its lounge section still a maze of plywood and furring strips. Luis Parada, in cutoffs and T-shirt, is relaxing, about to leave for the weekend; but Huki Land, in omnipresent green coveralls, is in the middle of a transfection and is just taking a break for one beer. About a dozen others are scattered in small knots around the large room, and appropriately enough the three of us are talking once again about the social aspect of a biology laboratory.

That is on Land's mind these days because by this time next year he will be in either England, Germany, or somewhere else in the United States, depending on which research prospects work out and which he decides to accept. "You have to socialize with people, to keep in touch with what's going on," he says. "That's absolutely important. It covers such a range of things, from simple ones like 'How do I go about doing that?' to major conceptual things, exciting new perspectives you get from talking with people. That's something you have to look for when you get to a place. How much day-to-day interaction do you get? The more the better. There is really a direct correlation between the density of people on the floor and the amount of interaction. It looks chaotic, but in the end it pays off.

"Our lab would not be our lab someplace else, and Baltimore's would not be what it is someplace else; it's all mixed territories. Here at the Whitehead there is something like a Baltimore space over here and a Weinberg space over there, but we're still together; and there's even been some talk of mixing everybody up again. The Fifth Floor," he says of the cancer institute, their first workplace already a historical phrase, "The Fifth Floor brought me the most exciting years I've had in science; it was a very special environment."

It's said by many people that Weinberg is good to work for.

"I always object to that phrase, 'work for,' " Land says. "It's not like a job where you work for somebody. You're part of it, the personality of the place. Sure, there's a group structure, and Bob is definitely the group leader and has the major responsibility, but the thing runs that well because people feel responsible for their stuff, and they feel it *is* their stuff. That makes the atmosphere really good."

Parada agrees. "I consider myself incredibly fortunate to have come here, and to have come when I did. I'm kind of spoiled as a scientist, getting used to what we've done here." Parada's next step, at least, is not the great leap of founding his own laboratory; one step behind Land, he expects to get his doctorate in the spring of 1985, then move on to Paris, where he will do postdoctoral research with the renowned François Jacob at the Institut Pasteur, one of the world's best-known biological laboratories. His work will focus on broader problems of development—that is, the organization and differentiation of cells as complex organisms grow, the broad questions for which cancer itself serves as a model. An intriguing notion, and Parada again points out, "Cancer research at this level really is not cancer research. We're molecular biologists, and we're interested in gene regulation. I sincerely believe that no one in this lab, including Bob, is fundamentally interested in cancer; we're fundamentally interested in how genes work, and cancer is a good system to study this. It's easy to assay [measure] for activity, and you have the feeling that the regulation of these genes is very important"—because of the multiple biological effects on transformed cells. "Because of the multiple, manyfold effects of transformation, this [field] is an interesting place to begin study. Yet what we've been doing has become the state of the art in cancer research."

An interesting symbiosis. The money came from cancer research toward basic biology because findings in basic research appeared important to cancer, and that proved to be the case. Now you can turn that around: Cancer turns out to be important to an understanding of basic biology.

"Exactly. And the majority of those grad students who have left this lab aren't in cancer research. But they are still studying gene regulation, just as they were; they haven't changed fields at all."

The caveat notwithstanding, both Land and Parada believe that these fundamental laboratory discoveries will provide the keys to treating human cancer—eventually. Parada says, "I really believe this work is going to block cancer from continuing to kill people, but that's years away. The fact that *ras* plus *myc* can cause a tumor has absolutely no impact on a doctor's ability to treat patients." Certainly a breakthrough from this research straight into treatment potential is possible at any time. "That would be a surprise. Of course, all this has been a surprise, but it would be too optimistic to expect everything to go like that."

And Land referred to the growth factors that he and others have been working to tie into cancerous, or neoplastic, transformation.

"I think about how you might cure cancer, specifically using growth factors," Land says. "If you know more about their action, you might take steps to control them. You might have very specific molecules you could use" to attack tumor cells, "instead of these sledgehammers like methotrexate. I think in five years we'll know much more specifically about these connections between growth factors and tumors. Someday I believe we'll see cancer treatment based on these discoveries."

Land's destination would turn out to be the Institute for Cancer Research in London. In the spring of 1985 he would tell me, "I'll be sharing some laboratory space with Michael Waterfield," who had discovered the homology between *erbB* and the EGF-receptor gene. "The best part is that there doesn't seem to be a problem with grants. Everything seems to be well funded."

16

The Meeting Ground

Tom Roberts's laboratory is in the Dana–Farber "Jimmy Fund" building, an adjoining structure named for a boy killed by cancer whose public fund went on to support construction of these laboratories and other center activities. Roberts is a genetic engineering whiz; to turn Luis Parada's phrase around, he has good hands. Long, raw-boned hands, the kind you would expect on an Indianan good at working on machinery. Lanky, mustached, soft-spoken, he is regarded as one of the world's best "cloners," somebody who can tinker with the invisible, complex, and temperamental machinery within the genes of bacteria until they tick along like the microscopic equivalent of a world-class sportscar.

Roberts was one of Lynn Klotz's top graduate students, "the kind of hardworking Midwesterner I used to always go after," when Klotz was looking for the bench scientists who would work at his lab at Harvard.

Roberts was later a postdoc in Mark Ptashne's lab at Harvard, doing some of the groundbreaking work in "overproduction of gene expression" in the late 1970s—in other words, arranging the strongest promoters and best binding sites within the genes of bacteria, splicing in genes of interest, and getting the bacteria to produce those genes' products in huge quantities. This was the kind of work, pioneered by David Goeddel of the genetic engineering firm Genentech, that resulted in commercial production of human insulin, a hormone, another kind of protein.

Roberts has worked in many different bacterial and viral systems but is now most interested in a virus called polyoma, a DNA tumor virus much like SV40. Polyoma is so named because it causes multiple tumor types in mice. The virus is favored by scientists like Roberts because some of the complexities that make SV40 sometimes nightmarish, if fascinating, are simplified here. SV40 has two "early" genes, so called because they are expressed early in the virus's reproduction cycle. Both genes are responsible for its ability to transform cells; one produces a large protein, the other a smaller one. Appropriately, with a small play on upper and lower case, these are called big T and little t.

Remember how genes are "read out": You travel along the DNA, beginning near the promoter and moving downstream, reading letters in groups of three: GTC would code for the amino acid valine of the resulting protein, AAT for the amino acid asparagine in the protein, and so forth. But the SV40 virus is extremely tiny—only 5,243 base pairs complete its DNA chain, a strand no longer than many single human genes.

Evolutionary pressure is the mother of invention: SV40 and a few other viruses that must fit the instructions for a lot of proteins on very tiny DNA strands developed ingenious "multiple reading frames." If one messenger RNA can read ". . . GTC–AAT–TCA–G . . ." then another messenger RNA can begin initiating gene expression at a different point: ". . . G–TCA–ATT–CAG . . ." One DNA strand; several sets of protein products. This is precisely the kind of mutation that can and usually does result in genetic disaster; in SV40, however, it resulted in getting multiple messages out of minimal space. But as James Watson has pointed out, multiple reading frames are not an evolutionary advantage in organisms with a lot of DNA to work with, because in SV40 and similar systems, a single mutation can foul up several genes, a distinct evolutionary disadvantage.

Polyoma virus has not two but three early genes, but although it has multiple reading frames, investigators can select mutants that distinguish these gene products. That is, they can select a strain whose DNA is mutated such that one early gene will be expressed while its neighbors on the overlapping reading frame will not be. The virus is about as small as SV40—5,292 base pairs of DNA. It has three sequences that were known to be involved in transformation: big T, middle T, and small t. The middle T has been known for some time to be the gene directly responsible for transformation, and its protein product is called middle T antigen. For now, antigens may be thought of simply as a class of substances that act against a host.

Roberts was now working in collaboration with Brian Shaffhausen of Tufts Medical School, a couple of miles north of Dana–Farber. Shaffhausen was the virologist in the team, the expert on polyoma virus, Roberts the molecular biologist. To explain the importance of Roberts's contribution to such a collaboration, remember that they are working in systems too small to be seen under a light microscope, whose components, so important to understanding their action and origin, can't be seen under any circumstances. But in a way, cloning and purification of genes and overproduction of their products are to biochemistry what supermagnification is to the microscopist: They allow you to get measurable, analyzable quantities of the chemical components of genes or proteins that in any given cell population would be too small to detect. For example, for the work they were planning, Roberts and Shaffhausen hoped to develop an antibody to middle T antigen. Antibodies can, for now, be thought of as antigens' opposite magnetic numbers. Antibodies attract and bind to antigens; antibodies are a way, then, of collecting antigens. In order to study them, antibody and antigen would have to be raised in quantity.

Here was the discovery that set Roberts and Shaffhausen on their course: In 1983 British scientist Alan Smith had discovered that in cells transformed by polyoma virus, the middle T antigen was always found bound to the protein of cellular *src*—the oncogene named by Michael Bishop, found in the Rous Sarcoma virus.

Here is a key point to come back to. The true oncogenes captured accidentally by viruses from cells are not normal genes. These viruses cause cancer quickly because the captured genes are mutant, transforming cells immediately. The normal cellular versions of these genes carry out tasks vital to cell metabolism. The *src* gene product, like that of *ras*, is found within virtually every animal cell. So important is its role, so strongly has it been conserved throughout evolution that it or a near cousin are found in organisms as primitive as *Drosophila*—fruit flies.

The *src* oncogene found in viruses had been mutated and caused tumors immediately in susceptible animals.

The *src* gene found in polyoma-transformed cells had *not* been mutated. However, its protein, Smith had reported, was bound to the middle T antigen. "As soon as he told me that," Roberts recalls, "I said, 'somehow the middle T antigen makes normal cellular *src* protein behave like mutated viral *src protein.*' So we set out to find out what middle T did to *src* that made it oncogenic."

Here might be a great key in the long chain—in fact, perhaps the chain was not so long after all. Perhaps Roberts and Shaffhausen could find how middle T changed an ordinary protein to send its activity haywire, toward cancer.

Down into the theater of the mind, one more time, to a level at once far simpler, more complex than before: the whole cell, the great earth globe of a cell before an astronaut's eyes, filling nearly the whole field of vision, the only thing illuminated in the dark.

At least now we can *see* the cellular membrane, the ribosomes within, the cellular nucleus; and at this magnification we can gratefully forget the DNA for the moment. Even the skeins of chromosomes are just tiny rods in the nucleus, little K and X shapes set within the nuclear sphere. At this level, though, we witness whole sea-changes in the cell's behavior without being able to see what caused them. This cell might suddenly begin swelling and dividing without giving us much clue why. Or it might change shape or shrivel up and die.

We need to back up to look at some tongue-twisting notions— the last tongue-twisters of this trip, and among the most valuable in showing what's really going on.

There's a physics demonstration showing how chain reactions work that has made the rounds of a few classes and science films. It is usually shown while someone is explaining atomic nuclear fission. Hundreds of mousetraps are set in a room, and on the trigger of each a Ping-Pong ball rests. Now you drop a Ping-Pong ball on any of the traps. It flies off and sets off at least two more, which in turn set four or more in motion, and within seconds the air is filled with clattering Ping-Pong balls.

It isn't chain reactions that are of interest here so much as massive reactions of particular kinds, but some of the imagery of that demonstration is useful. Imagine that in lieu of Ping-Pong balls we had different *kinds* of things set on hundreds of thousands of mousetraps. Imagine them in different colors and shapes—a thousand of this, a dozen of that, a hundred thousand of those—all quiescent. Now some single event occurs—a few white Ping-Pong balls come slamming out of nowhere and hit some big purple shapes; they just glance off, nothing happens. A few more Ping-Pong balls come flying in and hit some little red rectangles. Now *they* shoot off, each of them striking four or five objects as they go, but of the four or five they only *cling* to one of a particular kind, say, the green shapes, and now this bonded red-green thing bounces around and sets off some puffy yellow spheres—and now the room temperature is up half a degree from all that energy of motion. That elevation in temperature is enough to twist the huge purple things out of shape, which sets off *their* mousetraps, and into the air they go.

I haven't described anything particular here; just a little abstract three-dimensional theater. But when we talk about the behavior of molecules within the cell, we have to remember that there are usually anywhere from hundreds to hundreds of millions of copies of them that may be in the motions described. When we talk about the cancer pathway, we are talking about *one* cellular complement of DNA that may be sending out only several messengers to the ribosomes, but the action frequently escalates exponentially—in a kind of chain reaction among different kinds of molecules—so that in the end we may be talking about the actions of millions of enzyme molecules carrying out a reaction in the cell that then would be visible under a light microscope.

Earlier I was thinking about growth factors and growth-factor receptors, and how their alteration—mutation—might lead to cellular transformation. But seeing them schematically as little growth-factor plugs popped into receptor sockets doesn't tell much about how they work, nor about how they relate to the rest of the cell's sea of chemical molecules to interdigitate to and from the nucleus command center.

Lew Cantley is an expert at that. A biochemist, his specialty is cellular metabolism, the sort of thing I was trying to envision—the sea changes, tidal shifts that occur within the giant earth of a cell as the result of a small number of events at and in the cellular membrane. Like a weather forecaster of the cell, Cantley studies the changes in ion balances—the charged, incomplete molecules that sometimes trigger, sometimes foreshadow major events within the cell. And in the course of that he has had to spend considerable time studying enzymes.

Enzymes effectively determine the reactions that occur in cells. James Watson had summed it up succinctly.

Tightly controlled chains of reactions involving millions of molecules at a time go on inside the cell constantly. *Control.* The Ping-Pong balls inside the cell are extraordinarily specific, unlike those of the chain-reaction game; and the controllers of reactions are, virtually one and all, enzymes.

To make sense of what follows, it helped me to envision massive reactions of millions of different colored and shaped objects in Ping-Pong-like reactions. If someone referred to a molecule of enzyme A-ase interacting with B and C, creating B–C, I pictured the enormity of the reactions by envisioning one of these reactions beginning with a few enzyme molecules far below the visible, ending with what scientists call the phenotype: the observable biological behavior.

So Cantley will say, "Release calcium in cells and you see an immediate reaction." Indeed, "see" is just the right word here: You can observe it under a microscope, the combined effects of a few million doubled-up bananas (enzymes) hit by hundreds of wedges (enzymes) in a chain reaction that opens them wide. Once open, activated, the banana enzymes go to work flooding the cell with millions of calcium ions. We are talking about the chain reaction of one massive fleet of molecules scattered throughout the cytoplasm to the sudden entry of a fleet of a different kind, directly cause-effect. Some enzymes work slowly, but others can carry out their template-forming actions thousands of times a second.

The enzymes of particular interest to cancer researchers these days are of a class called kinases (kīn-āce), most often tyrosine kinases. Most chemical molcules are named for their components—calcium phosphate, for example, being a compound of calcium ion and phosphate ion. But enzymes are proteins that all *do* something, so most frequently they are called by their action name. *Kin + ase*: The prefix is the Greek word for move, the suffix a fairly universal enzyme-designator. Kinases are enzymes that take a phosphate group from one molecule (usually the cell's major phosphate-bearer, ATP), and donate it to another molecule. The "tyrosine" means that the method of action is to phosphorylate, or transfer a phosphate group, onto the amino acid tyrosine of the recipient protein. Serine–threonine kinases phosphorylate those amino acid subunits of proteins. The purpose of the phosphate donation is to activate the recipient molecule, itself an enzyme, or another doer-molecule.

It would be easy here to get lost in the loops of biology. Enzymes catalyze chemical reactions; often those reactions are to activate other molecules, and often those other molecules are enzymes, which may go on to do the same thing. This long chain of regulation is effective because the numbers of molecules involved as we proceed along the chain may move sharply up or down, or we may move from one series of reactions within the cellular membrane into the cell itself and finally into the nucleus, or vice-versa. It is not unusual for one tyrosine kinase to activate another tyrosine kinase, and so forth.

Cantley pointed out that adding a phosphate group to an enzyme or other effector molecule is one of the simplest and best methods of activation. Nature, therefore, uses it frequently. So it was with great excitement that cancer's basic investigators greeted a discovery by Cantley's colleague Ray Erikson in 1979, at the very beginning of the oncogene story. Erikson found that the protein encoded by the *src* oncogene was a tyrosine kinase. The next supposition one would make is that it phosphorylated some major regulator of growth to activate it; but which one?

Src's protein is in the cytoplasm of nearly every animal, as noted, so important is its (unknown at this point) function. Later, it was discovered in David Baltimore's laboratory that the *abl* oncogene was also a tyrosine kinase. Still, years would go by before further con-nections could be made, tying the oncogene proteins' kinase activity into the cancer pathway.

I mentioned the explosive changes that can be brought about in the cell by the up- or down-regulation of these enzymes to effect limited chain reactions. Let's look at the giant cell once again from two entirely different perspectives. First, look at the cell membrane as the film of a detergent soap bubble. In the sunlight you can see colors swirl and spin, expand and contract across the surface. Those whirling patterns on a soap bubble represent different molecules traveling across the cell's surface, normally long molecules with one end pointed out into the air, the other end pointed inward into the bubble. Some shorter molecules do not stretch all the way through the cell's membrane; they may point head-end outward, tail-end in, with similar molecules pointing head-end into the cell, tails also to mid-film. The cellular membrane is similarly constituted.

Watching the swirling motions of patterns across the surface, you are seeing not only the physical migration of some of these molecules around the sphere, but often their alteration into different molecules —that is, the chemical migration of molecules from form to form.

Among the constituents of this membrane are mortarlike molecules called lipids, as well as many proteins. The major lipid that would be of importance to Cantley was that impossible, singsong molecule mentioned earlier, phosphatidylinositol (PHOS-pha-TI-dyl in-OS-i-tol), hereafter (mercifully) PI. PI is phosphorylated to change it into other, more complex molecules in one of the most important of these chemical migrations in the cellular membrane.

Now, freeze the swirling motion and let's look at the cellular "traffic pattern" from another perspective: in a time slice, a stop-action picture. The cell membrane can be seen as a terrifically complex set of side-by-side, tightly packed arteries: some wide-open throughways that admit molecules or allow their departure, others like bundles of wires designed to admit information into the cell or send it forth. There is an enormous traffic of molecules into and out of the living cell, and each membrane constituent regulates its own type of traffic.

Or its own type of message. The growth-factor receptors, remember, are those information transmitters that generally pierce the entire membrane: head-end out for contact with growth factors, tail-end in to signal another protein. So far there have been several growth factors discovered, but the most studied and best understood are the aforementioned EGF and PDGF, insulin, and two forms of so-called transforming growth factor. Not surprisingly, these growth factors act in the most-studied and best-understood cell types— fibroblasts. Cantley believes that a wide variety of other growth factors may ultimately be found. And with them will come a nearly equal number of growth-factor receptors, most of them probably in the cell membrane. He expects that, like those already discovered, the receptors' outward-pointing head ends will be unique, each locking specifically onto its own unique factor coming out of the blood or connective tissue. The inward-pointing heads should be virtually identical, because the message they deliver within whatever cell they lock onto will be the same: Grow, divide, proliferate.

All the growth factor receptors discovered so far are tyrosine kinases. That is, the means by which they pass their message into the cell is by sticking a phosphate group onto their next contact. These "next contacts" are largely a mystery. Obviously they are important; they generate the appropriately named "second messengers," the number-two class of molecules in the relay race.

The membrane constituent PI can generate such second messengers, and that fact led Cantley down the interesting path he is on today.

We may be in the middle of a bewildering set of names and functions, but the chain reaction we are looking at is visually fairly simple. Out of the dark comes a growth factor (signal). It slams into its receptor, for which it has a chemical affinity. That changes the electrical balances within the receptor, so *its* shape changes. In its new form, the receptor is a perfect template for placing a phosphate on a nearby molecule. This is the first step in a branching chain of events leading to the critical second messengers for cell growth. Since the receptor can do this many times a second, the activation of just one receptor can cause the old Ping-Pong reaction: Millions of second messengers stream out, *into* the cell, as well as *across* the cell's membrane surface, their newly altered form making them active and able to carry out reactions on yet a higher scale. It's easy to see that within seconds, if we scale up the reactions logarithmically, we will see something. We will finally *see* something. And indeed, we do: The level of calcium ions in the cell will shoot up explosively, and the acid–base concentration of the cell shifts slightly in the direction of base—chemically, that means the pH of the cellular solution has risen.

Big deal.

Very big deal. Many of the enzymes at critical steps in cell regulation are known to be sensitive to sudden shifts in calcium and pH. Almost magically sensitive.

We tend to think of calcium biologically as a nutritionist would: as a building block of bones and teeth. Usually found in nature in chalky or stony form in combination with other chemicals, calcium to a chemist is a metal which, in solution, becomes a strongly positive ion, written $Ca++$.

To a student of developmental biology, however, the quick increase in calcium ion levels inside a cell is one of two major triggers of the even vaster range of chemical reactions ending in cell proliferation and in some cases even the development of a new organism. The second major trigger is a sharp increase in the pH, the base concentration, of the cell. Cantley believes those same signals may be used to control cell division in later stages of development.

By trigger, I don't mean these are merely indicators of something else going on, I mean they make all the rest happen. Consider the following experiment, simple in form, whose results are stunning to the layman and illuminating to biochemists like Cantley.

This experiment uses an intermediate cell in the progressive differentiation of female cells toward the egg cell, called the oocyte. In other words, the oocyte is not yet quite an egg cell, but it's headed that way. The oocyte contains half the female's total chromosome complement, as the egg will, the other half normally being provided by the father if the egg is fertilized. With the addition of calcium, the oocyte duplicates its chromosomes to complete the full set, a tip-off of the wonder to follow.

In the experiment, oocytes of a frog were extracted and placed in culture. No sperm were present: These egg-precursor cells were unfertilized. Now calcium was injected through a glass needle drawn microscopically fine, and the pH was hiked, marking an increase in the basic level of the cells. The oocyte now began to grow and divide. At the proper time the ball of cells began to differentiate and finally completed differentiation into a new frog—a tadpole—the exact genetic copy of its mother. Presto: one cloned frog. This is a "daughter" in the strict sense we associate with bacteria: the inheritor of all its single parent's DNA, a fatherless clone.

No magic, no other controls; just a sharp increase in calcium and pH, and all the machinery is turned on for proliferation and development—and if only in a frog, that at least offers a measure of the importance of increased calcium and pH.

Cantley was reflecting on the importance of these two events and their relationship to a second messenger he had been studying—phosphatidylinositol, PI. Its chemical migration into various related forms is called PI turnover, and within the past two years Cantley and many other biologists have become convinced that PI turnover is a major regulator of cellular metabolism.

The following discoveries were the foundation for that conviction, three linked events that enabled investigators to trace footprints back into the cellular membrane, to PI.

First, a particular kinase was found to have a major role in oncogenesis. It is called c-kinase; its composition is not relevant here. Japanese biochemist Yasutomi Nishizuka discovered that c-kinase, located within the cytoplasm, is the receptor for phorbol esters. Remember, those include the croton-oil tumor promoters so dangerously carcinogenic. Phorbol esters are so constructed that they virtually slam through the cellular membrane and latch onto c-kinase, activating it, and the cell becomes transformed. So far, so good. The next question is, naturally, if the way phorbol esters go about promoting tumors is by activating just one enzyme, c-kinase, what *normally* activates that enzyme?

Answer: calcium and one of the molecules in the PI turnover pathway. In fact, this molecule activates c-kinase by binding to it, changing its shape—just like the phorbol esters do. Fully two other, separate stages in PI's chemical migration sharply increase the release of calcium ions from intracellular stores. In turn the calcium steps up c-kinase and other kinase activity.

Thus, PI turnover appears to yield the normal regulators of c-kinase.

C-kinase, like an incredibly powerful switcher keyed on, rushes throughout the cell, phosphorylating other proteins that somehow, still mysteriously, regulate gene expression, and within minutes of the activation of c-kinase, the messenger RNA of a known nuclear onco-gene named *fos* comes streaming out into the cytoplasm to be trans-lated into its protein, its job unclear but its timing perfect—the cell is now quickly moving into its division stages. *Fos* is always expressed when cells are transformed by phorbol esters, but it is also sometimes expressed when growth factors are present.

Here was a beautiful place to stand, finally, for a clear view of one part of the oncogenic process: You could see the phorbol-ester tumor promoters short-circuiting a normally tightly controlled pathway, doing every time they slammed into the cell what other activators did only occasionally: turning on c-kinase.

Cantley: "It seemed clear to me that if PI metabolism regulates cell growth in such a major way, then some of the enzymes in its pathway should be regulated by [protein products of] oncogenes. The question was: which oncogenes?

"I was intrigued by a poorly understood enzyme that puts a phos-phate on PI. This reaction is essential for generating the second messenger for calcium regulation, and the enzyme is ubiquitous, from yeast to man. What if the tyrosine kinases—which have been implicated as essential for several growth-factor receptors and onco-genes, including *src*—evolved from PI kinases? What if they now function as regulators of the system?"

Enticing support for this idea came from studies of the viral *src* protein in a collaboration between Cantley and Erikson's labs at Harvard and from independent experiments by Ian Macara and his colleagues at the University of Rochester.

Lew Cantley had just pulled into the parking lot at Dana–Farber Cancer Institute to deliver a seminar when he ran into a hurried Tom Roberts. They knew each other well, but mostly from the basketball court. Roberts had been Lynn Klotz's graduate student and Cantley was a faculty member in the same Harvard department. All three were avid basketball players, so Cantley and Roberts had met often at the Harvard Law School gym. Now and then each heard a good word of the other through Klotz or other common acquaintances, but their work had little in common.

"Where you headed?" Roberts asked.

"To give a seminar."

"Can you tell me what about in one sentence?" Roberts was hurrying over to Tufts to talk to Brian Shaffhausen, his collaborator, the middle T antigen viral expert.

"I think cellular *src* regulates PI turnover," Cantley said.

Roberts stopped in his tracks. They exchanged a few words; their ideas after all had much in common. Though each of their approaches was radically different, at the moment that was the luckiest of breaks: Each had a different expertise. So they set about to test Cantley's point in a long series of experiments that, along the way, achieved a couple of firsts. Roberts managed to tune up cellular machinery to such a fine pitch that for the first time they were able to purify and collect large quantities of middle T antigen, the cancer causing protein of polyoma virus. Roberts developed an antibody that would act as a magnet for the middle T antigen.

And here is where they now stand, in a paper published in *Nature* in March 1985: "The complex of middle T antigen and *src* protein has PI kinase activity," Cantley says.

A long way from proving the last steps in the transformation of a normal cell to uncontrolled proliferation; but think of the simple picture it offers, if it can be proven. The *src* protein is the normal activator of that whole PI turnover that sets in motion one level of switches that in the end activates the Great Switcher: c-kinase. C-kinase rushes around the factory turning on machinery, sounding warnings. *Src* in turn is switched on *normally* by another still-unknown kinase, but only rarely, when cell reproduction is wanted. Abnormally, middle T antigen can activate *src*. And that's why polyoma causes cancer in susceptible animals. Just as calcium and one of those PI turnover products (diacylglycerol) normally shape c-kinase to do its many jobs—but latch a phorbol ester onto c-kinase, and the same thing is done, not at the right time, but at any time.

"There's a lot we still don't know about this," Cantley says. "But I really think we've taken steps in the right direction. We need to study more of the normal controls of PI turnover. And we still don't know how *src* normally is activated."

Completing the picture, consider the other improper pathways we can take to activating c-kinase. (See Figure 15). Add a growth factor

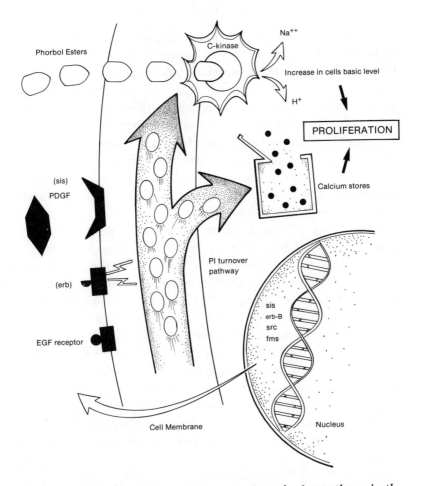

Figure 15. Most recently, scientists have implicated a key pathway in the growth and division of cells as the target of many oncogenes' actions. A major step in this pathway involves activation of the enzyme c-kinase (also called kinase-c). The pathway, called PI turnover, involves the combining and recombining of molecules, with each new combination signalling another growth step within the cell. Thus, some scientists now believe there are three related ways to activate the PI pathway and c-kinase: normally a growth factor (such as EGF or PDGF, pictured) latches onto and activates its receptor; one or more oncogenes (such as erbB or sis, pictured) may be activated, producing proteins that set this chemical migration in motion; or phorbol esters may be added—powerful tumor promoters known to activate c-kinase directly. Phorbol esters cause rapid tumor growth, yet do not mutate DNA, never even entering a cell's nucleus. Until recently, it was a mystery how they could cause cellular proliferation.

that has been over-expressed (PDGF, whose gene is very similar to the *sis* oncogene) to charge up the PI turnover in the cellular membrane. Truncate the growth-factor *receptor* in the membrane so that it signals for continuous PI turnover even when no growth factor is present (*erbB* oncogene is homologous to a truncated EGF receptor, which seems to affect PI turnover in some but not all cells). Or, most directly of all, send in the phorbol esters to accomplish directly what PI turnover does eventually: activate c-kinase.

And how remarkable that after all these years, we should still be looking at a marriage of chemical carcinogenesis and the viral model as the basis for understanding cancer.

Now Cantley tells me he heard a rumor from the Salk Institute at San Diego, but he is not sure where the rumor originated: C-kinase is the protein product of a known oncogene. Someone is pretty sure of it. So there might be another direct way of putting the cell into its transformed state: The oncogene for c-kinase may be mutated in such a way that it encodes for the constant production of c-kinase, or perhaps, in the cancer cell, oncogene c-kinase is mislocated by some form of crossover (translocation) so that it sits in front of powerful promoters that keep it expressing all the time. Or perhaps the oncogene is mutated so that its c-kinase is always in active shape, doesn't need another kinase or a phorbol ester to turn it on. There are so many questions to be answered here, but now, at last, it seems we have found the corridor down which we can locate those answers.

But what a long, winding road just to here: What all this supposed misregulation leads to, Cantley points out, is the production of a *benign* tumor, one that grows out of control but is frequently encapsulated and never leaves its home anchorage. What another researcher would call a glorified wart. So far I may have pointed out all the ways a cell proliferates out of control. But that's not what a doctor calls cancer. So far we have nothing to explain how these proliferating cells acquire the additional abilities to leave home, move out of their native tissue, and metastasize into distant colonies in completely different organs of the body from where they began. *That's* what cancer is.

17

Skyline

A late August day and I'm headed from the Whitehead over to Dana–Farber, to talk to George Canellos and Craig Henderson, then to the Harvard School of Public Health to visit John Cairns, both a respected scientist and a noted maverick in cancer research. And in the evening a short hop from the Longwood Avenue subway stop down to surgeon Blake Cady's home.

And thinking: Looking for certainty is not the same as looking for security, but there are resemblances. As we push farther and farther into the unknown we try to gather, grain by grain, bits of certainty that will transform the unknown to the familiar, the vague to the solid. The difference is that the hunt for certainty never gets comfortable, never quite arrives. On the contrary, there is a lasting discomfort here, like a continual demand on the muscles that leaves a residual fatigue; things never *finally* resolve themselves.

When we go from the laboratory to cancer-the-medical-problem, we encounter the same quandaries in only slightly altered form. True, there are no squabbles about what is or is not transformation; this is the world of cancer the killer. But Gulliver style, we escape a world too small to deal with, blow right on past daylight reality, and end up in a realm quite Brobdingnagian.

An easy trip: From the Whitehead Institute you can see, across the river, the Longwood Medical Area. Take the subway from Ken-

dall Square station, the train emerging from the darkness to cross
the river on the Longfellow Bridge, pass the Boston Science Museum,
change at Park Street, and finally alight at the Longwood stop, down
in a leafy bowl of trees with a stream rushing by—just a few blocks
from Dana–Farber and seeming a world away.

As the train crosses the river, look at the Boston skyline: as irregular an outcropping of buildings as you'll find in any big city. There's
a cluster of skyscrapers downtown, around the Park Street station,
each of radically different height but overall taller than elsewhere in
the city. Then scan south along the river: a lower profile, broken
now and then by a very tall building. (Dana–Farber is eighteen
stories.) Somewhere you might be able to dig up the number representing the average height of a Boston building; you might compare
it to the average building height in Los Angeles or New York. You
might compare the heights of various Boston buildings to the average
and nod approvingly if a given one checked out right on the average.
But what would such activity tell you that could possibly be of use?
Could you figure out the height of a given building by reference to
that average? It's as silly a proposal as trying to figure our chances
of getting cancer, knowing only that it strikes one in four. The
average is meaningless because each of our individual chances are
scattershot in clumps all over the place, with few of us *on* the average
and then by coincidence.

Virtually all the questions we laymen ask about cancer are based
on such simple-minded statistical averaging; yet the statistics, the
hard data, are of profound interest to medical scientists, and it is
some of those statistics I spent the day discussing, ending up now
in the evening touching on more of the same. Blake Cady and I sit,
feet up, beers in hand, on the cool porch of his home, the din of
crickets a constant background.

What's an epidemiologist? Someone broken down by age and sex.
What's a surgeon? Good hands, no brains.

Why are oncologists like fleas? They bug you constantly but don't
really do anything.

So the doctors in each specialty of cancer treatment jibe and poke
at one another, sometimes in good fun. Not always, neither between
specialties nor among many doctors of the same specialty-service in
a major cancer center like Dana–Farber. Blake Cady, surgeon, is

ruminating on some of the effects of the day-to-day contentions in hospital life after a long, hard day. Tall and slim with iron-gray hair, he sits with his bowtie loosened as we play devil's advocate with one other, trying to see through the fog that plagues newcomer and expert alike in trying to divine the secrets of cancer.

Cady has spent his twenty-year medical career in cancer surgery, beginning here in Boston City Hospital, working his hardest and most educational years at Memorial Sloan–Kettering Hospital in New York, moving back here. He is an intellectually restless man who not only loves being a surgeon, operating, but also loves the more tortuous, intellectually stimulating problems of fundamental biology. Not a common trait among surgeons. "Surgeons are by nature optimists and enthusiastic," he says. "They talk cases all the time. The cases are the fascination, and I think that keeps them from being bored without being too interested in fundamental biology."

Cady, because of his rigorous training in Boston and New York, had the opportunity "to report thousands and thousands of cases, and that's where you begin to be able to make real observations. The average doc in the community, or even in a hospital, will see only a few cancers and sometimes no rare ones. I've had the chance to report some very rare cancers, and after you do that enough—you have to do it—you begin to pick up on patterns that other people don't notice."

Cady and his wife, Bets, who is active in the cancer hospice movement, live in a spacious old home in a Brookline neighborhood close enough to the sprawling Longwood Medical Area to be "so full of doctors it's called Pill Hill." Blessed with a sense of humor and known for his graciousness to residents, colleagues, and patients alike, Cady has a reputation much like that of Emil Frei; yet, a colleague points out, Cady and Frei frequently disagree and are often seen by those around them as total opposites.

"Yet they're of very similar character underneath," the colleague said. "They both reason by anecdote, and both, when up against the harshest possibilities, would intervene rather than sit by and do nothing. Frei is a chemotherapist, and that's cutting edge, that's chic now; Blake is a surgeon, and that's out."

And, longtime resident of the medical community, Cady has interesting observations about that shift. He points out that over the past decade there has been a major shift in the leadership of cancer management (as the whole treatment process generally is called). Once the exclusive domain of surgeons, cancer treatment became the work of radiologists and then of those specializing in chemotherapy, medical oncologists. And it is the latter who have come to dominate the field, he says without rancor, "partly I think just because they have that tag, oncologist, which at the time [ten years ago] surgeons didn't have."

Now surgeons have also specialized; an organization of surgical oncologists has recently been formed. "You can see the change most plainly at hospital tumor conferences." Cady says. "Ten years ago tumor conferences were always led by surgeons, had been forever; now they're run by medical oncologists. Partly it's a fact of life— surgeons are busy in the middle of the day, their schedules are tight —but mostly it reflects a changing attitude toward what you can do." He sees a shift coming, not because chemotherapy is not useful but because he believes it has been overused.

"I saw a woman today, had a little tiny breast cancer, less than a centimeter in diameter, and no involvement of the lymph nodes"— that is, the least serious form of cancer, in which metastasis would not likely have occurred. "The medical oncologist wants to do a bone scan on her every six months from now on, permanently. Here you've got a woman with an almost 95 percent cure rate [with simple surgical removal of the tumor] and I had to say no. What are you doing this for? $200 a crack, $400 a year? Why do that? You know why? It's the technological imperative: We've got it so we've got to use it." The use of such costly high-tech solutions without evidence that they will help, Cady is certain, "is breaking the system; it's driving the system under."

Cady is not kinder to cancer surgeons, whom he sees tending to perform unnecessarily complicated operations over simpler ones "because the challenge is greater."

"Surgeons like challenges; if you can tell them they can do something that's a little more complicated, more challenging, they naturally respond to it and want to do it and find reasons why it's better." And he points toward the major debate going on now about breast cancer: So many clinicians are now claiming that less aggressive breast surgery is as successful as such extreme operations as radical mastectomy, in which breast, muscle, and lymph nodes are removed. His comments foreshadow the announcement by Bernard Fisher months later (discussed in Chapter 19). The same debate rages in thyroid cancer, where the trend has been toward total removal of the gland, Cady says, "even though the chances of complications in total removal are far greater" than in less severe operations that leave most noncancerous tissue.

Part of the problem is that everyone has numbers supporting his stand. Part of the problem, now, is that the sort of massive, long-term study of cancers that might prove or disprove a given approach are lacking. Without convincing epidemiological evidence—solid statistics over large populations—Cady finds himself buttressing his arguments with biological arguments against unnecessary treatment. "But sometimes your biological information is much less persuasive than the technical challenge, surgeons being what they are."

These are all reasons why people of equally good motives contend over proper treatment. In fact, the more "interventionist" doctors frequently call the more conservative physicians "nihilists," as though, in despair of anything working at all, they were willing to try nothing. But beyond that Cady believes a less honorable motive must operate as well: "There's no question that surgeons get paid more for doing one operation than another, so you pick the one you get paid more for—at some level that has to enter into it, and it's probably subliminal."

The problem, as Cady and many others see it, though, goes beyond the attitudes of doctors to the heart of American attitudes toward medicine, and it is here they find an impassable wall. "A woman comes in for a checkup after a tumor has been removed, and the doctor, by palpation, says that she is free of lumps. Then he does a mammogram and it shows her clear. 'Whew,' she says. Now that a machine has said it, it must be true."

Americans are beguiled by technology. It's interesting that the negative side of this fascination shows through every aspect of cancer: Laboratory researchers want few fancy machines between them and the submicroscopic world; physicans see false hope in the belief that some sort of machinery will end cancer.

Cady, for example, has a plan he believes would rid America of 75 percent or more of its most fatal cancers within a reasonably short period of time. It would involve large government expenditure but far less than is now being spent dealing with the disease: "A public education program that would get people to quit smoking or not start, that would wean people off high-fat meats toward lower fat, toward lower-cholesterol diets, would do more than medicine will ever do by intervention to lower the cancer rate."

Boring!

Lung cancer is the deadliest by far of the major cancers, and it is virtually entirely caused by smoking. Breast cancer had been the major killer of women until it was recently surpassed by lung cancer, as the surge in women's smoking thirty years ago finally took its toll; breast cancer that is not hereditary is strongly related to high-fat diet. Colorectal cancer, the third leading cause of death here, and stomach cancer, which takes a huge toll in the Orient, are both strongly related to fat and cholesterol in the diet. "People don't want to hear that," Cady says. "They want you to undo what they've done."

But it's not even necessary to consider diet's relation to cancer, which is somewhat tenuous, to see what physicians are up against: Smoking's link to cancer is solid, immutable, yet people keep on smoking.

Cady's words virtually echo those of George Canellos, chief of medical oncology at Dana–Farber: "Why can we cure Hodgkin's disease and not lung cancer? Perhaps because Hodgkin's disease involves the kind of series of errors you're talking about, that are being studied in the lab. And now someone comes through the door who has smoked himself to death for thirty years, bathing his lungs and bronchial tubes in poisonous, noxious chemicals every day of his life, and he's got emphysema and lung cancer, his heart is shot. He says, 'Doctor, do something for me.' What can we hope to do at that point?

"I suggest that the most common deadly cancers are those of older people, which may be the result of a lifetime of abuse, whether willful or not. It might be abuse by the environment, it might be dietary abuse of the colon, but if you smoke yourself to death and drink yourself to death, there is not much we can do."

Then isn't it surprising, on the other hand, that *everyone* doesn't wind up with cancer?

"That's a function of the body's amazing ability to repair itself,"
Canellos said. "But how much can you expect?"

And there is the doctor's ability and inability to repair, the frustration when sometimes efforts fail, the quandary the art of medicine
leads to, when doctors are forced to play hunches. Each interprets the
quandary in his or her own way, reflecting as many personality types
as there are doctors. But no one is immune from the tug of the case at
hand, not even when it tugs against the data—maybe especially
not then.

Craig Henderson, reflecting on the wide range of treatments at
Dana–Farber that are ultimately hammered out in conferences over
each case before a tumor board, repeats what he calls the two great
clinical fallacies: "One is that a bad prognosis justifies any treatment.
That is, if the situation is desperate enough, try anything but don't
just stand there. The other is that any treatment is okay as long as
it's nontoxic. They both stem from the same idea, and they offer the
doctor the same lure: 'I have to do something for the poor lady. I
cannot simply hold her hand and watch her die.' "

Medicine is still more art than science, a point scientist Michael
Kriegler would make emphatically and with admiration very shortly.
But even art needs its underpinnings, its forms. And for that medicine looks outward to the vast numbers of case histories that will offer
grounds for this treatment or that. And every doctor speaking on the
subject of statistics, epidemiology, the study of disease patterns and
spread, quickly comes to the same issue, says it the same way.

Henderson: "It's illusion versus reality. And of course you look at
something and you're sure it's not illusion; yet so often that's just
what it is." Example: "You look at patient A and you see the progress of a breast cancer to this point; it has spread to this point. So
you make a prognosis on what will happen. You now look at patient
B and see a quite different picture, so you make a different prognosis. But maybe you are seeing precisely the same course of development at two different times. And maybe when you think two cases
are identical, you're seeing two radically *different* cases at different
times, when their appearances coincide."

Now Cady and I are talking about the related case, in which a doctor is trying to determine whether all the cancer treatment developed over past decades has really improved survival, or whether doctors are simply seeing cases earlier and therefore imagining lives are prolonged. This is the lead-time bias referred to in Tucson by Hugo Villar—and ironically, when I mention his name, Cady recalls having just heard from him for the first time.

Lead-time bias: A hypothetical cancer kills all its patients ten years after the first clonal tumor begins. Twenty years ago we used to see it only in year seven, so for our five-year mortality tables it was 100 percent fatal. Now, with improved detection methods, we catch virtually all these cancers in the first year. Statistically, it looks like the death rate has turned around; in fact, nothing at all has happened.

For some of those cancers mentioned—those now deemed curable—it is known that lead-time bias is not generally influencing figures. But that cannot be known for all cancers, and while NCI gives out figures daily showing that one or another cancer's survival rates are improving, most of the doctors who deal with cancer every day are quite skeptical. Cady does see improvement in some cancers because of early detection—specifically in breast cancer—when cancers can be caught before they metastasize. But even here there is a caveat: Several cancers are now more treatable because they are being caught at earlier stages. But stage for stage there has been virtually *no change* in cancer mortality in forty years.

"In other words," Cady says, "if you have stage IV breast cancer, your chances today are no better and no worse than they were forty years ago. It's just that forty years ago more people got to stage IV and never had the chance to be cured in stage I, as we can now."

That is still good news for those fearing they may get cancer, to be sure, but it also indicates that most advances in cancer treatment are related to early diagnosis. Further, some radiation and chemotherapy protocols have their own mortality rates, some are known to lead to leukemia later on; they are given only to patients with virtually no chances of survival. Some particular kinds of bone marrow transplants have extremely high mortality rates, and there is heated dispute—at Dana–Farber as well as other centers—whether the hopelessness of the cases justifies this extreme intervention in which all of a patient's bone marrow is destroyed to wipe out leukemic cells. Success depends on whether the relatively small implant of new marrow can grow fast enough to supply the patient with new white blood cells and other key components of the immune system. Bone marrow transplant recipients are so immune-depressed they must live in completely sterile environments until they recover.

Cady extends his skepticism—which is to say his critical judgment —to programs he administers. He is in charge of the intraoperative radiation therapy program at New England Deaconess Hospital, a block from Dana–Farber. Highly touted only a few years ago, the idea of this protocol is to open a patient up on the operating table, then directly irradiate the tumor. "The rationale is sound," Cady says, since intense radiation can be targeted specifically to the tumor, minimizing otherwise severe damage to other tissues. Or, conversely, it enables the physician to administer more powerful doses than would be possible through chest or stomach tissue.

But success? "Totally unknown, really; I think it's another false technology," he says, borrowing a phrase from Lewis Thomas. Thomas speaks of true technologies, which emerge from an understanding of natural processes and prevent illness, and false technologies, which bring high-tech machinery to bear on a problem without preventing the problem. Says Cady of the intraoperative technique: "It's interesting to talk about and I'm enthusiastic in one way, but it's totally unknown whether it works or not. It may prove useful in a very selective situation; clearly it will not apply to a broad range of tumors."

Cady is concerned that the hope engendered by such experimental techniques may spur illusions—in the public, in cancer victims, in doctors—that successful treatment is at hand when in many instances it is not. He cites a famous case that was reported at Dana–Farber some ten years ago, a "foolproof" method of treatment. The case involved osteogenic sarcoma in children, a bone cancer with "a natural history so uniformly bad through time that everyone knew it could not change on its own." In a joint test, doctors administered an extreme chemotherapeutic regimen to children suffering from the usually fatal disease. After one year, they found a remarkable, dramatic improvement in cures and prolonged lives. Cady calculated that the cost of the intensive regimen was $300,000 to $400,000 per "life saved." The spectacular results of the study were published in the *New England Journal of Medicine*. Naturally, that set a precedent for this extreme and exorbitant protocol.

Then, a few years ago, the Mayo Clinic in Rochester, Minnesota, conducted its own trials of the protocols—randomized trials this time, a quite daring move given that the experimental protocol seemed to be working. In randomized trials, different groups are given different protocols, purely by random selection so that prejudgment will not enter into a given patient's being picked for a particular treatment. They found the same increase in cure rates no matter which of several treatments was followed. In other words, the expensive chemotherapy was no better than more traditional treatments, but for some reason this form of cancer no longer was as deadly as it once had been.

How had the original study gone wrong? Cady reflects, shrugs. "Suddenly, we had a case where the entire natural history of a disease changed before our eyes, across the country, for no apparent reason. But no one realized it because they hadn't done randomized controls. It hadn't seemed necessary." A disease almost uniformly fatal suddenly had responded to treatment—a variety of treatments. To this day no one knows why.

(Months later, evidence would be published to throw Cady's speculation into doubt but underscore his point even more solidly concerning the lack of finality of supposedly conclusive pronouncements: Two separate randomized clincal studies reported to the annual meeting of the Society for Clinical Oncology in Houston disputed the Mayo findings, tended to support earlier observations by Tom Frei and colleagues at Dana–Farber that the protocol against osteogenic sarcoma worked.)

Earlier that day, Craig Henderson had pointed to an even more famous and far more serious appearance of an artifact in epidemiology. Primarily in the early 1950s, women who had not been able to carry a baby full term because of spontaneous miscarriages were treated with the hormone DES, diethyl stilbestrol. It appeared to work, to enable many women administered the drug to have babies. "Appeared," because the entire topic was full of subjective pronouncements. For example, many women would miscarry many times and would then carry many babies to term without incident, without any treatent.

When randomized surveys were done, they uniformly indicated that DES was of no value whatsoever, that it was no more effective than placebos. "But many doctors continued giving the DES," Henderson says, an example not only of the delusions one can run up against when acting by hunch, but a perfect example of his "second clinical fallacy": Any treatment is all right as long as it is nontoxic.

DES, of course, proved to be a deadly carcinogen, not in the mothers who took it but in their female offspring, many of whom several years ago were found to develop an extremely rare vaginal cancer at a rate far above normal. "So the treatment was not nontoxic after all, but that's just the point. You can never really say with certainty that something is nontoxic. You don't use something unless there is solid evidence it works. The same old rule was operating, though: I've got to do something for this poor lady; I can't just do nothing."

And if doctors at Dana–Farber and other major centers have difficulty divining true from false technologies, Henderson said, consider the position of the physician in the community attempting to keep up with the latest in treatment. "By the time he sees the results of our trials, we may have rejected them, or we may be onto something entirely more promising. It just takes so much time to get the word out."

In a similar vein, Blake Cady now says, "I tell all my patients, for Pete's sake don't read anything about cancer in the newspaper. You have a combination of aggressive reporting combined with aggressive [searches for] funding and the enthusiasm people have to do serious research. There's not one percent of what's written about cancer in the newspaper that's still valid a year later. But that combination creates a lot of illusions, and they're pretty hard to overcome."

Looking for certainty, for some number to hang a hat on, some point at which the fulcrum, rightly placed, might move the world. Let's try one more shot: If the microworld is full of fuzzy lines and indistinct entities, and the macroworld is full of error bars and artifacts shimmering like mirages on the landscape, what happens when we attempt to pair the two? Can we hope to predict how discoveries in the laboratory will be reflected in improved treatment? Cady is fascinated by developments in oncogene science and molecular genetics but does not believe they will have a major impact on treatment soon, if ever: "I don't think cancer is that kind of disease, a disease like polio that you can prevent with a single blow."

Illustration. Cady suggests the possibility that all of us have microtumors, but that they only metastasize in a tiny percent of the population. "What do you do, tell people they have microtumors? Scare hell out of them for nothing?"

I suggest: What if we could identify a protein always expressed by a particular oncogene just prior to metastasis in breast cancer? In other words, what if we had a marker for metastasis that would be like a siren-alert to intervene?

Cady nods understandingly. "And then what? Screen every woman in the country? The financial pressures on medical care are incredible; they're breaking the system. You just aren't going to do something like that."

He points to a recent study at the Mayo Clinic. Longtime heavy smokers were brought in on a regular basis for bronchoscopy and intensive analysis of sputum. "They managed to detect lung cancer so early that the tumor couldn't be localized. What do you do for these people now? You know they have cancer and you can't find it. That's worse than not knowing. If some day it turns out that there's tissue specificity for given tumors, you might find a hot spot by scanning, but if you try to drive things back too far, you wind up with insuperable problems, financially and technically."

And Cady cites one of his favorite pieces of clinical advice: "Don't look for things you don't want to find."

When we say a tumor metastasizes, we mean that a cluster of the tumor cells—let's say liver cells—migrates into the bloodstream or lymph system and settles somewhere else, like the lungs. New tumors arise. Are those tumors of lung cells, induced into cancerous behavior by the migrant colony, or are they colonies of the originals continuing to grow?

"The original tumor cells! Yes, that is amazing," Cady says. "You can look at a metastasis of the lung under a microscope and see liver cells there. People will say, 'You haven't proven smoking causes lung cancer; Grandma died of lung cancer and she never smoked a cigarette.' Well, lots of times cancer in the lung was what killed her, but that was a metastatic tumor colony that had originated in the breast or somewhere else."

The liver is an even more common site for metastatic migration, which could easily make the connection between drinking, say, and liver cancer appear doubtful by introducing false-negative connections: examples of people with liver cancer who had never drunk alcohol.

Finding certainty in this "real world" is no easier in the end. Witness: Cady recalls a case when he was a resident at New York's Memorial Sloan–Kettering. "A woman had had a very small breast tumor twenty years earlier, less than five centimeters, no evidence of metastasis. Now there's an outbreak of hepatitis in her apartment building. Hepatitis, as you know, damages the liver in some way that makes it a target for liver cancer; most liver cancer is found in populations with high rates of hepatitis. Several of the cases in the building presented with clinical hepatitis, others just had symptoms.

"The woman had the classical symptoms of hepatitis. She was a smoker, lost her taste for cigarettes; that's one of the symptoms. Admitted to the hospital. Urine turned dark, and she came down with severe jaundice. No matter what we did for her she went rapidly downhill, died in three days. Initial cause of death was hepatitis.

"But at autopsy it was found her liver cells had almost entirely been replaced by breast-cancer cells. Twenty years later! Explain that to me. *She had cancer cells no place else in her body.* Somehow, twenty years earlier her breast tumor had metastasized to her liver, before it was removed from her breast; but the cells had lain there, inactive, whether controlled by the immune system or simply dormant, who knows? What had the hepatitis done to set them on their way again? And so rapidly."

We sit silently, the crickets' vibrant storm of music rippling back and forth across the dense foliage of late summer. Finally he says:

"Somehow a balance had been upset. I think about that all the

time when I hear about metastasis. That it isn't just automatic, that
it doesn't seem to be a single simple thing—certainly not in that
case."

And yet, to Cady and others, despite the frequency with which
events can confound our attempts to put numbers on diseases and
their treatments, we are overlooking numbers that are hard and re-
liable, and it is time for them. They are easy to come by and full of
surprises. We avoid some of the solidest, perhaps because we don't
like the look of them. They are the numbers that relate some cancers
to smoking cigarettes and other uses of tobacco, and still other cancers to diet.

John Cairns is a believer in those numbers. Though they approach
cancer from different perspectives, Cairns's and Cady's views seemed
to me to be closer than those of any others interviewed. Cady is a
surgeon, Cairns a molecular biologist (he is also a physician but has
not practiced for many years). Cady's real world begins and ends
with the reality of a scalpel; Cairns, as he talks, constantly pulls out
books, journals, or papers from his file drawers. He is a bibliography
sprung to life: late fifties, spume of curly white hair, very British, his
face now and then twisting with the droll humor of some point,
some irony; fond of irony; and at each question or each statement
suddenly moving to a book so that his citation of articles becomes
quite literal. "There now, you see," pointing to the constant number,
the chart with its deceptively steady curve. Moving on to some new
point and in motion: to the file cabinet from which he will pull
the article in question, dropping it in his visitor's lap.

This, in fact, is one of the things he says he does these days, "more
or less acting as a reference point for others." He is the well-known
author of one of the best books on cancer for the general public, a
probing look at how we see cancer and how we fail to, compressed
into the slim *Cancer: Science and Society*. Now nearly ten years old,
this book has proven quite prophetic.

Writing in 1974 through 1976, Cairns forecast that the next decade
would see little change in mortality from the most fatal cancers, and
he suggested there would be no major treatment improvement that

would extend life significantly. He predicted there would be no widely applicable cure found. And finally, he predicted that screening would not prove generally feasible even if it was helpful in limited cases. Other than the Pap smear, "other screening programs haven't had spectacular success even though the medical profession has tried to get them, because, of course, it's a wonderful way of turning out business. Still, people don't go for it, and indeed it is not clear that it does very much good."

In the evening, Cady noted that the single diagnosis of breast cancer really covers two separate diseases. It occurs in young women, and here there is a hereditary connection but no apparent relation to diet. It also occurs in postmenopausal women, and then there is no hereditary connection but a strong relation to fats consumed and to obesity. Many doctors resist calling both diseases by the single name breast cancer. Then why do so? Because the cancerous cells under the microscope are identical; out of apparently unrelated causes, a single physical disease appears to occur.

Cady noted that if a screening method for the first type could be found that would enable doctors to tell a young woman she was at "70 percent risk," they might be alarming her and forcing changes in her lifestyle without knowing whether the advised changes would really have any preventative effects.

Cady: "So what if we had a screening method for the first type, and we could tell a young woman, 'Instead of being at average risk, you're at 70 percent risk. So have your first child young, stay skinny, and if you're under fifty have regular checkups.' You could do that I suppose; it would be of no harm. But if, likely as not, it turned out to be a cancer for which you could do nothing in advance, set no life-style or eating habits that would help prevent it, you might be doing these women an enormous disservice."

In effect, you would be managing their entire lives from a very early age, based on predictions made from family profiles.

"And consider how that differs from, say, a Pap smear. Here we have a very limited region of the epithelium of the uterus involved. It usually occurs in women past forty and therefore past childbearing years. So if there's a problem, you cut out the uterus and you have prevented trouble. That is a very favorable case, and you're not likely to find another like it among the major cancers." In fact, the breast cancer that is the major killer among women is the postmenopausal, possibly diet-related variety.

No connection between diet and cancer has been made that is nearly as solid as that between smoking and cancer, but diet correlates remarkably well with kinds of cancers over large groups. Cancer rates vary radically worldwide, as Cairns has detailed in his book, and new findings are regularly reported in other publications. Colon cancer is virtually unknown in Africa; so is coronary artery disease, both so prevalent in this country. Africans eat virtually no fats, have very low cholesterol levels. Stomach cancer is a major killer in Japan; it is virtually unknown here. One can go on and on, spotting countries, correlating cancer rates. Are some of them hereditary, indigenous to that ethnic group? Few. The best evidence against that is the Japanese case. Japanese who move to the United States but retain their ethnic way of life have stomach cancer rates identical to those who remain in Japan; those who move to the United States and "westernize" have the same low rate of that cancer as any American.

Is industry and its certainly noxious pollution responsible? For some limited cases, perhaps, but not for the big numbers. If that were the culprit, Cairns notes, "you should look at nations that are not industrialized but are Western in every other way and find low rates of the major cancers we suffer. But look at Iceland and New Zealand, perfect cases in point, no difference whatsoever. You can look at a Seventh-Day Adventist, vegetarian family living in an industrial suburb next to a two-pack-a-day smoker and lover of marbleized beef, and the smoker will have the lung and colorectal cancer while the Adventist family will not."

Of course, Cairns is speaking metaphorically. In any given case either family might have cancer or be free of it; one unit is not a statistic. But that is not the point. The statistics have neat and skinny error bars. The view is quite clear: Clean living can go a long way toward preventing cancer. Of course, I would mention to Cady, this leaves out one critical element: American rambunctiousness. Americans do not wish to be told what to do. It is not merely that we, like everyone, look hopefully for someone or something else to blame for our problems, something that can be given a neat techno-logical fix; it is also that we are ornery.

Cady and I both have a good laugh on that bit of epidemiology. Cancer prevalence among the ornery. Cady says, "The kind of people who came to this country came because they couldn't stand it around the people they were living with." "Or couldn't be stood by them," I say.

Cady: "And when you look at our hospital and see the trouble we have with our own quit-smoking program . . . Hell, if it doesn't work here, what's the hope? Half of all nurses smoke, and there's even a percentage of doctors. Oh, don't get me wrong; the sociological problem I talk about is enormous, mind-boggling."

And Canellos had pointed out: "Look, the only significant *group* to quit smoking has been doctors, but that should tell you something. I used to smoke a pipe myself, had to give it up; had to. And I think you will find that catching on."

I had left Canellos this afternoon, headed from Dana–Farber to the Harvard School of Public Health, where Cairns's laboratory is, still in the Longwood Medical Area, with one stop to make in be-tween. Down the elevator into the lobby where patients and their relatives sit, waiting for treatment or waiting for someone to finish, or just waiting. Looking for the Dana–Farber public information office. It's across the parking lot, the guard points. Where? There. Where—ah, that old house? Right. A big ramshackle old Victorian decked out in gingerbread, the gingerbread perhaps a trifle moldy. But inside, redecoration is going on. Boxes lie scattered; an arrow directs me upward. And now here I am with an information officer. We are talking about where to find what. She is, all the while, half-visible behind a cloud of blue smoke, chain-smoking unfiltered cigarettes.

And a few weeks later in Washington, at the National Cancer Institute, somewhere in this holy of holies an information officer and I talk, excitedly, of the promises and the problems for the future in cancer treatment and research. Engrossed, she chain-smokes ciga-rettes. Filtered. I bum two. What else is new?

18

Gullywasher

The world of cancer research is small, as I've said. Mention someone who's done something of note and the others, certainly those in the forefront, will know of him or her. The world of cancer treatment is considerably wider; still, the top doctors in a given specialty will know of the others. Mike Kriegler is one of the few people with wide acquaintance among both groups—not a situation he would have elected, but he wasn't given the choice. He was a student in Lynn Klotz's class at Harvard, was a classmate of a friend of Cantley's we chatted with one afternoon in early summer, was a classmate of Karen Antman—who is now an oncologist at Dana–Farber—was a patient of George Canellos.

1975, and Mike Kriegler, twenty-three, is a graduate student in molecular biology at Harvard. His special interest is development; he has always been fascinated with the enormous chasm between the single-celled organism and the more complex: Somehow a cell takes energy and materials from the environment and organizes *itself* into a complex organism. But like many young people he is certain of little beyond that, rotating from laboratory to laboratory trying to find his niche, the special magic of the right mentor, the right project, the right colleagues.

It's November, a chill, gray time in Cambridge, and he comes down with the aches and pains and chills of flu, so it's off to the Harvard Health Center. Flu it is, they tell him, and among the usual remedies of rest and fluids someone there suggests a hot toddy. Now he develops more severe aches; by early January he is totally debilitated and in constant pain. He gets chills and fevers in the night, and finally he passes out cold.

An x-ray discloses a figurative "water bottle" enclosing his heart, water having filled up the pericardial membrane that surrounds the heart. The symptoms are all typical of (a) tuberculosis, (b) heart disease, (c) lymphatic cancer. *If I'd gone to a cancer specialist, he'd have seen cancer. If I'd gone to an infectious disease specialist, he'd have seen TB. But I saw a cardiologist, so he saw heart disease.*

Kriegler lies in a hospital bed as residents and interns are paraded into his room to peer at chart and subject: a classic case of endo-carditis. Two weeks later he is, in the worst sense, upgraded: thromboma—very, very serious. A surgeon opens a window into his chest to withdraw fluid and there sees the final answer: a huge lymphatic tumor clutches Kriegler's heart.

February 1976, his twenty-fourth birthday, Kriegler is on his back with Hodgkin's disease. There are a lot of ways of staging the severity of Hodgkin's. You can be A, with a lump, or B, systemic, and the tipoff to B is what are called circadian fevers; they come on schedule, with sweats in the night. He is B. You can be in stages I through IV, with IV being most severe, depending on how many chains of lymph nodes are involved. He is a III. And you get a final letter E if there is involvement below as well as above the diaphragm. On this one he lucks out; he's just a IIIB. How curable is Hodgkin's disease? *Obviously a IIA is more curable than a IVBE. And there's the art of it, the incredible art of treating these diseases: How far can you push the bone marrow down with radiation and chemotherapy before you kill the patient? How much do you let the white blood count drop? How much of what drugs do you give? It is Art with a capital A,* says Kriegler the scientist.

Kriegler's system is administered bombs: intensive radiation followed by six months of agonizing chemotherapy, more radiation, another six months of chemotherapy. He is in hell, but he has lost none of the combative sense of humor for which he is known. One day a friend, Harvard Professor Jack Strominger, comes to his hospital room and asks if he's thought about his specialty, about what he'll be. *Look, I don't even know if I'll be a twenty-five-year-old.* But Strominger presses a book on him: *The Cold Spring Harbor Symposia on Quantitative Biology/Tumor Viruses. Eureka. That kicked it for me, that did it. Some people may be cynical about this, but until you've been there, baby, you really can't appreciate it. There's a lot of glamour and a lot of glory in this subject right now, but believe me, that won't have been a bad thing if it all works out.* And finally, Kriegler is taken off his chemotherapy and goes out to change the world. Spring 1977.

Summer 1984, plowing water northward out of Philadelphia. Rain comes down in sheets and waves tearing banks of earth, lifting pieces of macadam from the roads, leaving slashes of mud beneath the water streaming everywhere. Lightning and thunder had flashed and exploded through the night, without letup, and by morning buses, trucks, cars are plowing along water-filled roads like speedboats, sending six-foot waves in great gullwings to obscure the roadway completely, swerving past drowned cars and trucks. Finally: Fox Chase, the adjoining suburb known for its medical facilities, namely today the cancer institute, where Michael Kriegler has just begun setting up his own laboratory.

"I guess you could say having cancer got my attention, having cancer sucked me into it," Kriegler says, grinning. His humor is wiseguy: toward himself, competitors he disagrees with, even more with those promoting nonsense and quackery as cancer cures. "But there was something else. I wanted to help people; I wanted whatever I did to be of some use to somebody. I mean, I'd be dead right now if a whole bunch of brilliant people hadn't given everything they had to keep me alive. I wanted to pay something back."

It was the medicine, or the Art, of George Canellos, Rita Kelly, and George Rosenberg of Dana–Farber Cancer Institute that kept Kriegler alive. But he is not a medical doctor, he is a cancer researcher, one of the few who has seen cancer from as many perspectives as anyone has found. He is setting up his fancy digital DNA synthesizer. He is interested in molecular genetics as the main thoroughfare into the world of development—the idea that caught his interest in the beginning and which he never lost.

And isn't cancer, the negative imprint of the picture of development, the best place to learn? "Sure. I hear people talk about normal development; that's what they want to study. And I say, 'What's normal development? Can you define it to me?' And of course they can't."

I'm reminded of the postulate in linguistics that the second most important word in language is the equivalent of "no": the first is "yes," because as you're looking around you and trying to relate what you see, you need to be told you are correct; and then you need to know the limits of each word and description, and that means "no."

"Yes, there is one thing you can say about cancer for sure: it is *not* normal development. Now, if we can understand all that cancer is, all that *not*-normal development means, maybe we'll know a lot about what we mean by normal development."

Kriegler is especially interested in viruses, and in the future—perhaps even the near future if his work proves out—he envisions tailor-made viruses that might carry a "good" gene into the DNA of someone with a genetically damaged organ to effect repair. "Viruses, after all, are specific. A herpes virus will attack nerve tissue every time. It never makes a mistake. A hepatitis virus does its work in the liver. Why? Instead of trying to reinvent the wheel, we need to look at the way nature already has learned to do things and imitate that."

Playing nature: "It's incredible what you can do with this tiny collection of cells, of viruses—you know what a virus is? It's a piece of a cell. I mean, you look at it and say it's floating off on its own. But there's really nothing there you wouldn't find in a cell. It's just a piece of a cell, whether it started like that or not.

"It's like Tinkertoys. My favorite toys as a kid, and here I get to play with them all I want."

Except you can't see the Tinkertoys. Microworld, the world of those who build these constructs in their minds, cobble them together as Weinberg says, then wander from room to room.

For his own part, Kriegler thinks that too much of the unusual behavior of human cancer is being left out as Weinberg and others try to clear away the messy genetic jungle to get at its essentials.

"How about latency? An individual can develop a tumor, go into treatment for a year, go into remission for five years, and then recur with the same disease. There's something fundamental going on that we have no appreciation for. There are a few tumor cells left, and the immune system obviously is dealing with those cells, but then some event triggers new growth. It gets the upper hand, and cancer takes off again."

Again. Kriegler is free of Hodgkin's disease for just two months in 1977, then relapses; that's dangerous. The rule of thumb is that it's harder to get someone into remission after the first relapse, harder again after the second, and so on. He is put back on a course of chemotherapy, which ravages his system. Back to hell: He is given injections of the highly toxic nitrogen mustard, vincristine, and vinblastine.

Once cancer patients are established on chemotherapy, they become outpatients. Kriegler reports to Dana–Farber once every ten days. Although doctors monitor his case, he does not see them often; a nurse administers the assigned drug through an injection. His reaction is quick and devastating. Within twenty minutes he begins vomiting, and when his stomach is empty he continues with dry heaves for as long as eight hours afterward. He is completely debilitated. Some of the drugs make him feel like his veins are on fire. He loses his hair, but that is the least of his worries, and, despite the doctors' attempts to mitigate these side effects with one trial drug after another, including marijuana tablets to combat the nausea in an NCI trial, the pain and vomiting continue. Finally, a combination of tranquilizers and the powerful painkiller Percodan restores his equilibrium. Luckily, *I don't have an addictive personality; I don't know why, but I can take this stuff without ill effects.* Luckily, too, because through this period he will continue going to his lab every day to do his graduate work. Students and colleagues visit him during the periods when he's hospitalized, and he falls in love with one of them.

Mike and Marcie are married. She graduates and then begins studying for her MBA. *I go in and get my injection, and by the time I'm in the taxi I've got the dry heaves. I go home and continue, and with Percodan, I'm back in the lab the next day. But, you know, some of my best scientific work was done then. God, I wonder sometimes how anyone could go through cancer alone, if you didn't have people*

*around who cared for you. If you were just on your own I don't know
how anyone would have the strength.* And at last, remission again.
Now Kriegler is shooting determinedly at forever: no more, cured,
nothing.

The Krieglers move to Berkeley, where he takes a postdoctoral
fellowship in Michael Botchan's laboratory. (He remembers his time
in Berkeley, only just ended to come here, as a period of fine science.)
Marcie finishes her MBA and goes to work for Bank of America,
working her way up to a solid position. Usually when Hodgkin's
victims relapse, they relapse fairly quickly. Get to five years without
relapse and you're usually out of the woods. Rule of thumb. Kriegler
goes two, three, then four and four-and-a-half years.

In December 1982, Kriegler wakes in the night, bathed in sweat.
*It gets so you dread going to sleep, wondering if you're going to
wake with night sweats. But you can't let that get to you. You have
to put a stop to that. It can break you, it really can break you.*

To Sanford University hospital for yet another round of chemotherapy. This time his reactions are not so severe, and the combinations of painkillers keep him on his feet—and that in itself is a great
relief from apprehension.

"In effect I can live a normal life and probably will," he says. "I
relapse, I get treated and am better, I relapse again. The thing is, if
they can consistently do away with those side effects, that takes a
lot of the dread out of the thing. It may be that more and more
tumors become treatable. That even in the absence of a cure, people
will lead fairly normal lives as their cancer is managed"—an echo of
Jordan Gutterman, from what seems now years back when I interviewed him in Houston, on the development of tools (like his interferon) to manage cancer, and an echo of what many physicians at
cancer centers see as the eventual demise of cancer the demon: not
abolition but management. If we can't kill the beast, maybe we can
at least cage it.

Kriegler draws two general lessons from his bouts with cancer.
"You are not a statistic. There is no statistical measurement of an
individual case; statistics apply to large groups. For a while there, I
was scared, like everybody is. I said, 'What are my chances? What
are my odds with this kind of disease? What are my odds as a IIIB?'
And my doctor told me the most important lesson I learned then:

There is no way you can calculate odds on an individual case. If the disease is 90 percent fatal, you will not wind up 90 percent dead. You will either live or die. That's a yes or no, there's nothing in between. If the disease is 10 percent fatal, you get the same answer: You will either live or die, 100 percent of you. What is useful to an epidemiologist or an oncologist is not useful to the patient. Marcie was thinking of changing jobs when we moved here, and I asked her why, and she said she had just read that oh, 90 percent of new MBAs leave their first job after two years. I said, 'That's a reason? That's a reason to leave your job is you fell into a statistical group?' Statistics are not motives. I'm not sure what moves the world, but it's not statistics."

Lesson Two is more universal among cancer's survivors, put in a variety of ways: "I now appreciate the true value of time, the reality of it. You can't replace time, but while you've got it, it's yours. I don't want to waste any of my time. No baby steps, no sitting down and thinking what I might do that'll look good or that would be safe. I haven't made a name for myself, don't get me wrong; I have yet to make any great discoveries, but I think it's important that one tries to do great things. If you fail, you fail. What else is new?"

Outside the rain has stopped, the skies have cleared; it is a golden afternoon so hot, the air so drenched with water, it is hard to breathe. What else is new?

19

A Sure Thing

"The lady came into my office having had two mastectomies a year apart. Now she was frightened about the possibility of recurrence and had been given contradictory advice about what course of treatment to follow."

Craig Henderson, who heads the breast clinic at Dana–Farber, reconstructs:

" 'What should I do, Doctor? God, I am so confused. My first doctor said I should be given CAP [a common anticancer regimen], then I went for a second opinion and this doctor said I should have a year of Temoxafen, and finally a third said I should have a year of CMF. What should I do?'

" 'My advice to you is: Do nothing. I would go out and enjoy life to the fullest. I would assume you are cured and forget everything you've been told.'

" 'Now I'm more confused than ever!'

" 'Ma'am, there are no data here, there are no facts, there is no science here! I give you my intuition, as each of the other doctors did. You don't want that: You want my science, and rightly so. But there is no science here. Science requires empiricism, science requires data, science requires experiments. I can tell you about cases we have profiled by the hundreds: What does it mean to have two cancers rather than one? Lots of data on that. You had chemotherapy a year ago because your lymph nodes tested positive for cancer. I can easily extrapolate; there are reams of data on such cases, controlled experiments.

" 'But here is your case: You had two mastectomies a year apart, with a year of chemotherapy in between. How many cases fit that profile? I have none in the literature. Here is one with six years between mastectomies; here's another with two years. Are they relevant? I have no idea. No such data exist. So I advise you intuitively. My intuition is to trust nature until you know that intervention will help. If I were to say that this is scientifically sound, I'd be betraying science, I'd be dishonest. I'm giving you my *a priori* gut feeling about your case, but that's all I have.' "

But Henderson believes that in the effort to be sympathetic, to *do something*, oncologists around the country are pretending such intuition is scientifically valid. "Somebody tries something, it works; next week everybody is doing it. I think we're doing more harm than good with practice like that. Fifteen years ago cancer patients had nowhere to turn; no one wanted to treat them. Now there are three thousand medical oncologists and the country is full of radiotherapy palaces. It's a multibillion-dollar industry. Fifteen years ago drug companies didn't want to invest in development of anticancer drugs. Now they're making millions on them. I think it's sad the number of doctors we've trained, and how we've let the financing of medical education rest on cancer treatment."

Enter Bernard Fisher. Consider the thrust of his work against the background painted by Henderson. Of all the medical scientists in the country, none is more respected than he, and few are as influential. The head of the National Survical Adjuvant Breast Project (NSABP) in Pittsburgh, Fisher literally has turned around the course of breast cancer treatment for millions of American women over nearly three decades.

Fisher is a cancer surgeon who has the trust of the medical community, ranging from other surgeons to medical oncologists. Henderson describes the reputation of Fisher and his Pittsburgh group as impeccable.

He is a careful scientist, constantly harping on the need for good scientific procedure in determining courses of treatment for cancers

—especially the breast cancer that has been his life's work. Fisher's right-hand man, Norman Wolmark, is a biochemist as well as a surgeon, a very unusual combination.

Probably no group has been nearly as influential in turning breast cancer treatment away from the Halsted radical mastectomy, which had been introduced in the 1890s, to more moderate treatments such as the "lumpectomy" than has the NSABP with Fisher at the helm. This was not because Fisher had premonitions that the Halsted was too extreme, but because he was willing to challenge the radical procedure at a time when it was considered the only sure way to treat breast cancer, and to measure the efficacy of the Halsted radical mastectomy against less-disfiguring surgery, and then to track the success of follow-up treatments of every sort including the boldest of all —no follow-up treatment whatsoever.

The hardest thing to do is to do nothing. Few doctors are sure enough, or perhaps more accurately, are willing enough to admit the validity of their *uncertainty*, to test their own treatment theories against the ultimate control: no treatment at all. Yet that is precisely what Fisher has done at the NSABP for the twenty-five years he has headed it—included a no-treatment control in his randomized studies of breast cancer therapy. Politically such a protocol is explosive; should no-treatment prove as effective as the physician's chosen course of action, that demonstrates the physician has gotten nowhere; should the chosen course prove demonstrably better than no-treatment, the physician can appear a callous, inhumane number-cruncher denying effective treatment to a whole group of patients.

In a world of patients seeking positive thinking, optimism to allay their worst fears, such randomization of all groups of treatment protocols can seem a confession of weakness, of uncertainty. And so, of course, it takes the largest measure of strength to carry out such protocols in the face of real uncertainty.

Of all the U.S. science and medical journals, perhaps none is more powerful than the *New England Journal of Medicine*. Published weekly in Boston just a few blocks from Dana–Farber, the *New England Journal*, The Journal of the American Medical Association, and the British *Lancet* generally are regarded as the world's most influential medical journals. In Henderson's words, "A single lead article in the *New England Journal* can make one's reputation as a

scientist forever." It is influential, more importantly, in that a new
way of treating a disease or a new perspective on disease, when noted
in the *Journal*, often becomes the latest word on the subject within
days.

Bernard Fisher, the major force in breast cancer treatment, had
summed up virtually his life's work in two important articles sub-
stantiating that the Halsted radical mastectomy was *not* the treatment of choice in breast cancer. His conclusions were drawn from
publicly funded studies—protocols covering years-long periods paid
for by taxpayers through NCI and by charitable donors through the
American Cancer Society. The studies were presented in companion
papers submitted to the *New England Journal* in March 1984. Odd,
then, that six months later it seemed this preeminent force had met
an immovable object in the *Journal*: The articles remained unac-
cepted, yet unrejected. Few doctors concerned with breast cancer
were not buzzing about the lock-hold of the papers within the offices
of the *New England Journal*.

Cancer Letter editor Jerry Boyd responded angrily when asked if
he knew of the delay: "Holding up an article for peer review is one
thing, but there doesn't seem to be an excuse for this kind of delay."
As is often the case, that the NSABP article was delayed at the
journal was a poorly kept secret, unpublicized but known throughout the cancer establishment. "This is a publicly funded study,"
Boyd noted. "It was paid for largely by NCI funds. The public has
a right to the results of it."

What was happening? The normal course of events when a paper
is submitted to the *New England Journal of Medicine*, as with most
peer-reviewed journals, is for editors to ship the article to two reviewers. The intensity of review by peers can vary greatly from
journal to journal, and at the *New England Journal* the scrutiny is
indeed intense. However, it usually takes a few months for editors
to agree that among the dozens of articles submitted for considera-
tion, a particular submission does not merit publication in the Journal, at which point it is returned. If the reviewers split in their opinion, staff editors review the submission, as they do if both reviewers
agree that the article *should* be published. Changes may be ordered.

But that was not the case with the two submissions of Fisher and
the other NSABP investigators. The articles simply vanished within

the *Journal's* offices. If they were being peer reviewed, no one could find out by whom.

With so many influential doctors and scientists wondering about the course of those two submissions, it may seem odd that the story of the delay did not become public—that at least one of the interested physicians would not have gone to, say, the *New York Times* and opened up public inquiry. After all, these were studies whose conclusions would affect the course of breast cancer treatment for millions of women.

Someone might have done so, were it not for the Inglefinger Rule. To recap: Any article whose contents are discussed in any other publication will not be considered a candidate for publication in the journal. The aim of the rule is to prevent findings from being sensationalized in the public press before they can be laid out in their clearest, most scientifically careful form in the journal. It is a rule fully subscribed to by some doctors and scientists, hotly disputed by others who see it as a way for the *Journal* to give itself a profitable edge, an enforced "scoop" on other major publications. Nevertheless, in this case no one wanted to jeopardize publication of the papers in this most influential journal by blowing the whistle.

Further, the *New England Journal of Medicine* is usually reasonably fast in publishing, according to several oncologists, and that, combined with its authoritativeness, makes the rule seem generally a good one. What better vehicle for twin articles summing up the careful work of decades? Yet even thoroughness could not account for a delay that now had eaten up six months and that would, in fact, continue for a full year.

To understand the doctors' frustration at the delay, and Fisher's own, we have to go back to at least 1958, when Fisher became involved with his first clinical trials. The concept of the clinical trial is of paramount importance in cancer and *medical* science, and it is significant that Fisher described that relationship in a 1982 talk to the Society for Clinical Trials, of which he is a founding member. Fisher became involved in the first NSABP clinical trials to evaluate breast cancer patients undergoing a variety of different treatment regimens because his mentor "told me that I *had* to participate."

Fisher confessed, "At the time I had no interest in clinical trials, no interest in chemotherapy, and looked upon the whole endeavor as a distraction interfering with my laboratory investigations. Little did I realize that I would shortly reject that thesis and would become wedded to the clinical trial concept."

And little did Fisher realize that he would lead a team of scientist-doctors who would soon hypothesize that the breast cancer treatment of choice of this century, the Halsted radical mastectomy, was no better than some others. At the same time he was becoming aware that the "art" of medicine practiced by many physicians needed to become a science of medicine, less informed by the prior case handled by a given doctor or by treatment vogues or by "populism"—a word used by Fisher as a strong pejorative—and more informed by experience, by the same kinds of careful observation that underlay all scientific endeavor.

"Early in my medical career I was appalled at the 'willy-nilly' fashion by which treatment regimens slipped in and out of popularity. How many operations was I trained to do or medicines that I was instructed to give because of somebody's conviction that they were beneficial, passed into oblivion for no apparent reason, only to be replaced by others of equally dubious worth? Worse yet, how many countless patients have received those operations or have taken the medications?"

Fisher saw salvation ahead and, he said, like a true believer was certain that everyone would see it virtually immediately. "I became obsessed with the notion that the introduction of prospective randomized clinical trials into clinical medicine would surely make order out of chaos or science out of art." Each word in his descriptive phrase is vital. *Prospective* means forward-looking. In other words, unlike epidemiologists and other statistical analysts, his team would not be looking backward over the natural history of a disease and trying to infer what 'would have happened if . . . ,' or trying to draw conclusions about the efficacy of different treatments based on how they appeared to have worked in the past. *Randomized* is the element considered most important by those administering clinical trials. Those selected for various protocols must be picked from the eligible population purely at random. The physicians do not know which protocol is better; they must not pretend they do, or give in to hunches that determine which treatment their own patients get. *Clinical trials*: real people with real cancer, broken down only into allowable subgroups that reflect different disease behaviors. For example, in Fisher's major trials that we're now looking at, he made a distinction between premenopausal and postmenopausal women, because breast cancers always have behaved radically differently in these two groups. Further, he distinguished between women whose armpit lymph nodes tested positive for spread tumors and those who showed no such spread.

"Here was the opportunity to apply the scientific method for clinical problem solving," Fisher said. "When properly employed such trials could undoubtedly provide definitive information relative to the worth of therapies prior to their widespread use on populations as a whole."

Fisher had many unkind things to say about medical students' training in basic sciences, where he found lack of respect for the scientific method, and in clinical medicine, whose principles he found "antithetical to the clinical trial process."

Medical students "were taught to be individual decision makers and to treat patients according to their clinical judgment. They were unprepared to accept the concept requiring that they treat their patients according to a predefined protocol that selects therapies by randomization and gives them no chance to exercise their own decision making—which is more often than not related to the experience they had with their last case."

It was Fisher who pointed out that cancer treatment has historically been based on how the disease was seen biologically—regardless of what physicians might say of its clinical presentation and their empirical testing from that moment. And how cancer was seen biologically was usually a function of whatever biological "world view" was hot at the time. Thus, he noted in a 1980 article in the journal CANCER, by the second century A.D. the Roman physician Galen had already classified cancer as a systemic disease—but he related it to an excess of "black bile," one of the so-called humours believed to regulate bodily functions, and *therefore beyond the reach of surgery*. Thus, in a stroke, the centuries-old treatment of cancer by surgery reached a hiatus that was to last some 1,600 years, until the eighteenth century.

By the middle of that century Italian and French surgeons were writing articles claiming that breast cancer was a local "obstruction" that could be removed successfully, and they even recommended removal of axillary (armpit) glands as a safeguard, a procedure followed to this day.

It's worth noting now, when the Halsted radical mastectomy has fallen into such disrepute, that Fisher, the man largely responsible for turning medicine to alternative measures, gives no small amount of respect to William Halsted, the nineteenth-century surgeon who began treating breast cancer by removing breasts, underlying muscle right to the chest wall, lymph nodes, and often extended musculature. And for good reason. The simple removal of tumors, sometimes including nodes, had already been in practice since the eighteenth century, and the cancer invariably recurred. It was Halsted who suggested the radical—in two senses—operation that left women maimed and often partially immobilized, but often permanently cured them of cancer.

Henderson and Canellos wrote a major piece for the *New England Journal of Medicine* in 1980, surveying the results of various breast-cancer treatments. Though they ultimately point up the brighter future now faced by women with breast cancer, they say near the outset:

"No results, whether measured in terms of the percentage of patients free of recurrence (89 percent) or the percentage of patients alive 10 years after diagnosis and treatment (60 percent) have been better than those achieved by [Dr. C.D.] Haagensen in a series of over 1,000 patients treated with [Halsted] radical mastectomy between 1935 and 1973. On the basis of these data it is difficult not to accept radical mastectomy as a standard with which all other proposed therapy should be compared." (The authors move on to conclude that indeed better treatments have been discovered, citing the work of the NSABP.)

At the same time that Fisher explains the biological errors in Halsted's view, he chides current medical practitioners for failing to see that only by understanding the true biology of cancer and its spread can doctors hope to improve on Halsted's record. True, after citing the extraordinary record of radical mastectomy, Henderson and Canellos were able to write, "The argument that all forms of therapy should be compared with the Halsted radical mastectomy is no longer tenable; a number of less radical and less deforming treatments are at least as effective in achieving good local control, and changes in surgical practice are beginning to reflect this."

But the key phrase is *local control*. To understand the significance of the emphasis on local control by surgery, we have to look back to Halsted and the biological presumptions underlying his approach, as outlined by Fisher, and to understand that Fisher's first real evidence that the Halsted radical might have an alternative came from discovery of a chink in Halsted's *biological* presuppositions.

Here is how Halsted saw the spread of breast cancer: First, a primary tumor develops and grows. It grows outward by physical extension, eventually spreading beyond the breast into the lymphatic system, that pipeline of cleansing fluids paralleling the bloodstream. Within the lymph nodes tumors spread by extension much as a plant grows, new cells budding out from the existent tumor into the nodes. The nodes help block passage of tumor cells. Thus, finding involvement of lymph nodes is a measure of the extension of a single tumor body, like a plant spreading outward from its roots. Halsted further believed that the bloodstream was of little importance in tumor spread, and that a tumor was fully autonomous of its host tissue.

The key to Halsted's view from a treatment standpoint was that cancer's spread was linear—by extension—and orderly. Thus, removal of all the spread *local* tumor was the best that could be accomplished medically. Recurrences, Fisher noted, were considered failures of surgery.

By 1965–67, Fisher said, the NSABP was building considerable evidence that breast cancers do not spread in an orderly fashion, that metastasizing cells could move from bloodstream to lymph system and back again with ease, that in fact the involvement of lymph nodes was only an indicator of the extent of the disease, not at all a literal marker for how far it had traveled.

And those biological perceptions led in turn to the first major conclusions drawn by the Pittsburgh group, although not by them alone, and those conclusions are stunning in their reversal of traditional cancer orthodoxy. First, tumors metastasize virtually independently of the type of local control exercised by the surgeon, and second, most breast cancers have already metastasized by the time they have been located; that is, like leukemia, breast cancer is systemic, system-wide almost from inception. Thus, for example, an absence of tumor cells in the nodes is an important predictive factor as to whether tumors have metastasized and taken root *anywhere* else, for the nodes themselves are sites of metastasis, not merely of direct-extension growth of the primary tumor.

The companion articles by Fisher and other NSABP investigators eventually published in March 1985 reported:

• Ten years' results comparing radical mastectomy (Halsted) with total mastectomy, with and without radiation. Total mastectomy involves removal of all breast tissue but no underlying muscles, and is therefore far less disfiguring and not disabling. In this study, begun in 1971, disease-free survival was compared in women who had had the Halsted radical and women who had had total mastectomy. A further breakdown compared women in the total mastectomy group who had had armpit nodes surgically removed and those who had had radiation therapy to the nodes instead.

Results: No differences were found among women who had had radical mastectomies, total mastectomies with node surgery but no radiation, and total mastectomies with node surgery and with radiation. In other words, they concluded, rather shockingly, "The variations of local and regional treatment used in this study are not important in determining survival of patients with breast cancer."

• Five-year results of a separate randomized clinical trial. All patients had had breast tumors not larger than 4 centimeters—just over 1.5 inches—in diameter. Some had positive, others negative lymph nodes. All patients with positive nodes received chemotherapy, on the assumption that their disease was certainly system-wide. Now the randomized group: Some women were given total mastectomies, having all breast tissue removed but no removal of underlying muscle as in the Halsted. A second group got segmental operations or lumpectomies; within this second group some women got radiation therapy, others did not.

Results: With or without radiation, women receiving lumpectomies did as well after five years as women receiving total mastectomies. More surprising: With radiation, the lumpectomy patients did better than total mastectomy patients.

Most people hearing these results have the same reaction: What else is new? Lumpectomies have been the dominant breast-cancer

operation for more than a decade, gaining more and more acceptance among doctors. Next, why·the big delay in announcing the
results? What major impact could they have had a year earlier?

Fisher himself provides some of the answer to the first question in
a scathing attack on those who follow treatment fads without looking at the biology underlying such treatment—even if the treatment
be his own. In his talk to the Society for Clinical Trials referred to
earlier, Fisher said that in 1971, without a trial having begun on his
alternative hypothesis to Halsted's, "it seemed as if merely starting
the trial was catalyst enough to change surgical practice. Whereas
in August of 1971 one could barely get enough surgeons to participate [in NSABP trials] because they wouldn't do anything but a
radical mastectomy, by 1973 or 1974, when we . . . had no results,
surgeons doing radical mastectomy were few."

Should these new trials, then just under way and only in 1985 reported in the New England Journal, "demonstrate that radical mastectomy is not any better than a lesser procedure it will bring forth
a 'so what else is new?' If radical mastectomy should be found to be
better, the trial will be scoffed at, criticized and condemned. Not
only have surgeons long since given up radical mastectomy but they
are already two jumps ahead. They have become convinced in the
marketplace by American women, the news media, and a host of
important radiation oncologists unencumbered by firm data that
lumpectomy and radiation therapy is the treatment of choice."

Because of "that public relations approach," said Fisher, "that
wonderful clinical trial mechanism is endangered by those who practice the philosophy put forth at the trial of the Knave of Hearts" at
which the queen advises the jury, 'Sentence first, verdict afterwards.' "

Does all this, perhaps, represent the frustration of an overly pedantic investigator—too enamored of the science, too little respectful
of the art of medicine? Certainly not in the view of such believers in
the medical arts as Craig Henderson. It was Henderson, after all, who
emphasized the importance to doctoring of being there, of relating
personally to the patient, of offering a presence that in itself might
be healing and at the least could be comforting.

Yet in their New England Journal article, he and Canellos noted,
"These are difficult times for a clinician treating breast cancer, since
the conventional forms of therapy often become unacceptable before

new approaches are shown to be worthwhile. Furthermore, early widespread acceptance or rejection of a new technique may preclude adequate evaluation and precise definition of the role of a new approach." Both this article and Fisher's many writings close with strong optimism, foreseeing a near day when women will be given far more individualized treatments based on huge quantities of data predicting the behavior of more and more particular breast cancers.

But such data, to Fisher, can come only if the requirements of the randomized clinical trial are respected and clinicians as well as government funders do not leap to back unproven fads.

In a talk to the American Society of Clinical Oncology in San Diego in 1980, Fisher stated an attitude toward the basic investigator that could have come from a scientist most remote from the clinic:

"I am concerned by the hostility directed toward the investigator from all fronts, particularly if he/she should be so unfortunate as to be productive. . . . The peer review system needs modification. Its support of defined research projects rather than people and its posture as an adversary will ultimately weaken the medical and scientific eminence of this country. The self-serving politicizing, pressurizing, and downgrading of others which is related to disciplinary chauvinism and, more often than not, to a lack of . . . vision is antithetical to scientific principles. We must invest not in surgical oncology, radiation, or medical oncology; not in clinical or basic research; not in community physicians; not in cancer centers; but in talented people."

When the companion pieces were published, Fisher appeared in a joint press conference with Vincent DeVita Jr., NCI director. Both insisted that delays in publication had occurred only because reviewers had questions concerning the conclusions and the use of data that they wanted shored up, a time consuming process.

Nevertheless, Fisher later told me that such delays were becoming commonplace and were creating "a crisis in medical reporting." He did not want to discuss his thoughts concerning this particular delay, other than to say it left him as frustrated as it had others.

"In an era of instant (news) telecommunication, a 14-month delay is absolutely ridiculous," he said, "It creates a vacuum to be filled by rumor-mongering supermarket throwaways."

20

The Best Defense

In the late summer Lynn Klotz and I met several times at the house of his friend Ann Henderson and her daughters, Rachel, 17, and Mary, 10. Rachel was in and out, like most teenagers, had just returned from studying drama at Oxford and was about to begin her senior year in high school. A few weeks later—right now, early September, as I head south, ultimately for the NCI—she realizes she's been feeling very tired lately. Maybe an iron problem; unconcerned, she ups her iron supplements.

September fifth she, her boyfriend, and Mary head to the Boston Science Museum, but as the day progresses she feels worse and worse. At first tired, then as though she'd had sunstroke or some kind of heat exhaustion. Now she knows she has to see her doctor, Barbara O'Neil. The doctor believes Rachel has mononucleosis and runs a blood test. Just after arriving home, Rachel gets a phone call from O'Neil: Her blood-platelet count is drastically low—300 when it should be 300,000. Either Rachel's immune system is destroying its own platelets, an infrequent side effect of mononucleosis, or the platelets simply aren't being produced, the major sign of leukemia. She must report to Beth Israel Hospital over in the Longwood Medical Area immediately.

Home alone, scared, Rachel packs up and heads for the hospital, is met there by her mother, who is a psychology professor at nearby

Simmons College. Doctors take a bone-marrow sample, a procedure Rachel remembers as extremely painful. But by the next day, deliverance: Rachel has mononucleosis. It will take her weeks to recover, but there will be no lasting effects.

A few months later, a good friend of Rachel's comes down with the same symptoms of mononucleosis with a critically low platelet count. She assures everyone there's nothing to worry about; she knows what the results will be. But she is wrong; she has leukemia. She must leave college and eventually prepare for a bone marrow transplant, the ultimate, most severe treatment for leukemia that will not respond to other therapy.

Epstein–Barr virus causes mononucleosis in the West, is associated with Burkitt's lymphoma in Africa. What is the connection? Is one virus causing a leukemialike mononucleosis in Rachel Henderson, leukemia in her friend? Or is something else at work?

A little cooperation, please. It takes at least that much to keep traffic flowing on the highways, buses integrated in the stream with cars, aircraft obeying their patterns, pedestrians staying off the freeways and vehicles off the sidewalks so that even when traffic in the nation's capital jams up as it does for the better part of each workday, it doesn't stop altogether. And throngs are able to file down escalators into the Metro, thinning now as the train smoothly slides into each station, and departs, headed outward into the Maryland countryside cool with autumn.

Imagine once again the cooperation it takes to keep ten trillion cells humming along, differentiating just so, dying on time, being cleaned out of the system by cells under the same instructions; from a distance (far enough to see yourself in the mirror) the ten-trillionfold cooperative effort seems infinitely well coordinated.

We have looked down at one cell, more and more closely examining its controls at the submicroscopic level reachable only by the imagination (though what the imagination conjures can be shored by experiments), pulling back to see the sea-change affected in the planetoid cell, pressing down yet again to see one kinase activate a thousand, those thousand activate a few million, the millions create an effect visible under the light microscope—visible! Witness: The planetoid is growing, its nucleus swelling, the chromosomes multiplying, now drifting to opposite poles of the nucleus; the cell as though blurring becomes a double impression and finally splits into two cells, the two into four, the four eight, sixteen, thirty-two. A little math tells you that on the fifth division one cell becomes thirty-two, and by the tenth it becomes 1,024. All together now: 2,048, 4,096, 8,192, 16,384. In the computer age we might say that at division ten, we get a kilocell; at division fourteen, sixteen kilocells; and finally, somewhere around division twenty, a megacell.

Looking at cancer so far we have been just about this simplistic in imagining the tumor growing within the body, and we had to keep that view simple in order to range over the complexity of changes leading to that multiplication. Now consider this: The human body is not only under terrific controls from within the DNA command center, it has another whole level of controls in the immune system. We have to step back from that growing ball of cells to look briefly out at that system, because it seems certain now that cancer represents not only loss of control at the genetic level, but loss or defeat of surveillance by the immune system, a complex intercellular network that routinely rids the body of everything from its own dead cells to infectious invaders.

The first time through the NCI, I was thinking of viruses, hearing how learning their secrets brought new knowledge of the operation of living systems vastly more complicated. This time through it will be the relationship of the immune system to cells of one's own body versus foreign organisms, and it turns out that viruses are an interesting place to begin here, too. But we will look at viruses as attackers now; not as strings of genes that now and then turned out to mirror our own, revealing secrets of oncogenes, but in the way we ordinarily encounter them, as invading organisms seeking a host in which to reproduce. How do they work? Why don't they always work? Why doesn't the process of viral infection lead, like the mathematics of cell division, to the virtual explosion of the host with billion-billions of viruses?

Answer: Defense.

Everyone who has caught a cold has had an intimate association

with at least one and probably several RNA viruses, viruses that are
so simple they don't even contain DNA, but the related RNA. The
cold is caused by what is called a rhinovirus. Flu is caused by any
one of a family of RNA viruses, and we know that viruses cause polio,
mononucleosis, a wide range of cancers in animals, and at least one
form of leukemia in humans—the HTLV virus Robert Gallo would
soon explain to me.

A review: At most a virus is a piece of DNA enclosed in a protein
coat. It infects only tissue types specific to its own particular identity,
and it does so generally by slipping through the cell's membrane.
Once inside, one of two things happens. At one extreme, the simpler
viruses invade the cell's nucleus, the protein coat breaks open, and
the viral DNA is incorporated with the host's DNA, somewhere
downstream from a promoter. Now, if things go right for the virus,
whenever nearby genes are read out, the viral genes are read out as
well. New viruses are produced by the host's own genetic machinery,
along with new protein coats. They either bud out from the cell surfaces or, if they are so-called cytolytic viruses, when enough viruses
have formed they burst the cell wall, killing the host cell, and then
flood out into the surrounding tissues.

At the other extreme, the viruses may bring into the host most of
what they need for reproduction. They may need only the host's
ribosomal machinery, carrying into the cell the codes for many of
their own enzymes. These viruses simply send their own messengers to
the host's ribosomes to produce the viral proteins.

However alien viruses may sound to the body's well-tuned operation, few are even dangerous. Host defenses grow increasingly sophisticated as you move up the evolutionary tree. In humans, the most
basic antiviral defenses involve immunoglobulin—antibodies, proteins encoded by genes.

Viruses, like any foreign invading microorganisms, have surface
markers that identify them—much the way invading aircraft might
be identified by surface markings and silhouette. Antibody-producing
cells constantly circulate through the blood and their surface markings chemically recognize a particular antigen's surface markings, in a
lock-and-key fashion.

When an antibody-producing cell hits a viral antigen, genetic machinery turns on within the defender cell that produces antibody specific to the invader's surface markings in a lock-and-key fashion. *Completely specific*: One antibody generally matches one and only one invading antigen. Generally, the antibody protein produced in the defender cell latches onto the invading antigen, forming an insoluble complex that simply sinks out of the bloodstream. The more invading viruses—or bacteria, or other antigens—are reproduced, generally the more antibodies against them are secreted by the producing cells. The symptoms of most viral infections—fever, the rashes of measles and chicken pox, congested chest, watery eyes—are actually either part of the defense or the result of the antibody attack against the invaders. Ultimately, with most infections, the antibodies win. You get better.

Some viral protection is better than that. Often, once an antibody is mounted against an antigen, it remains activated for long periods of time. That is how vaccines generally work: Doctors introduce dead viruses or replicas of viral surface antigens into the bloodstream, mounting the antibody defenses in advance so the invaders never get the chance to multiply. Sometimes this early production of the right antibody lasts for life, as in the case of polio vaccine.

Certain antibody-producing B cells are present at low levels at birth. As the immune system develops, a "library" of antibodies is produced, each specific to a single antigen. The library offers an array of defenses against a wide range of possible antigens that might be encountered, each frequently in a single copy. When an antigen appears that is specific to one of these antibodies, the cell producing it begins expressing the antibody more rapidly. And then it begins reproducing itself as rapidly as possible. This way it can overwhelm the invader by producing antibodies faster than, say, a virus can reproduce. Then the B cell must shut down.

An interesting analogue to the cancer pathway we've been studying. What if the B cells don't shut down? Is this a way a virus might be "associated" with cancer without causing it? In fact, that may be just the connection. Most recently, scientists have begun to think that Burkitt's lymphoma, associated with Epstein-Barr virus, is only initiated by the viral infection. However, because of a promotion action, the B cells do not shut down. Other lymphomas may develop similarly. Although this is speculative, it suggests a direct explanation for how Rachel Henderson, infected with mononucleosis by E.B. virus, simply recovers, while a friend infected with the same virus develops leukemia, a cancer of the immune system.

There are other connections to cancer. First, at least some tumor cells have surface markers that distinguish them from all the other "self" cells of a person's body. The immune system is known to operate against tumor cells in at least some cases. Remember Shelly Bernstein's suggestion: Because chemotherapy kills cells by percentages, it is presumed that *some* tumor cells remain to be cleaned up by the immune system—which it sometimes does. But why "sometimes"—why not always? Why is the metastasizing microtumor not knocked out of action in the bloodstream?

There are many cancer specialists who believe that microtumors are commonplace, that the loss of control that leads to proliferation is so simple that it probably occurs frequently, that therefore the difference that leads to cancer such a tiny percent of the time lies in the immune system's not working properly in cancer victims.

Immunologist Vicki Sato had mentioned one day that during the early 1970s, there was a theory popular in the field that the true evolutionary purpose of the immune system was to check the spread of migrating tumors. The actions of the various immune-system components against viruses, bacteria, and various parasites was thus seen as "sort of an afterthought, a secondary function." And there is a lot of common-sense appeal in this idea.

First, diseases characterized by decontrolled, proliferating cells can be found all the way back through the evolutionary tree to plants, which can develop crown gall tumor and various similar explosions of growth. But metastatic cancer is not found until you reach fairly complex levels of development—about the level of sharks, immediately before development of the vertebrates. Set that fact aside for the moment and consider that after the fertilized, one-celled egg has replicated just five or six times into a blastocyst of thirty-two to sixty-four identical cells, the cells begin to differentiate. As differentiation proceeds, daughter cells are no longer identical to the parent that gave rise to them; though they contain the same DNA, all the same genes are not being expressed at a given time, or perhaps at all. The first such series of changes marks the differentiation of the blastocyst into endoderm, mesoderm, and ectoderm—inner, middle, and outer layers of the organism. There is a correlation, noted earlier, between these three and inner-organ, skeletal, and skin tissues. Nevertheless, during this developmental period millions of cells must migrate. For example, epithelial cells, which are relatively primitive and undifferentiated, are found in the walls of organs ranging from the stomach to the skin; but all epithelial cells begin in the fetus in the same group of barely differentiated cells. At some point, some of these cells migrate to the developing stomach, some to the liver, others to the surface of the fetus to give rise to skin.

At this stage, if the immune system exists at all it does not interfere with such migration. It seems reasonable to suppose that the immune response to migratory "self" cells develops later to pronounce a "stop," to hold the organs in place. In other words, if in early stages of fetal development massive migrations must occur, the problem becomes, how can such migration be stopped? The immune system's development might be the answer. Although Sato still finds the idea inviting, she believes it is probably oversimplified.

Here are the two major features of the cells of the immune system: They recognize virtually all other cells of their organism as "self," they are that generalized in their recognition pattern. And they recognize cells from other organisms, even of the same species, even of the parent or offspring, as "nonself," so individualized are they. How similar one person's cell markers are to another's is a measure of how closely related they are, but only in identical twins are such markers identical, and that is why organs are naturally rejected after transplantation except between identical twins. To prevent rejection in other patients, doctors must suppress the immune system, now leaving the patient at high risk of infection.

The collective immune system sounds like the true colony of cooperative microcreatures that each of us is in many ways. First, "macrophages" circulate through the blood and lymph, literally devouring cells that need to be cleansed from the system. They are scavenger cells, cleaning up not only invaders but such carrion as dead red blood cells. In another category are the lymphocytes, the white blood cells, consisting of B-cells and T-cells. Although the derivation of the names is not particularly important here, the differences in the cells' behavior is.

In ways still largely mysterious, all three cell types work together to elaborate the antibodies. In addition to the antibody response—that magnetic latching between antibody protein and invading pathogen—the T-cells mount their own direct response. So direct, in fact, that they are referred to as killer cells. The combination is an array of defense cells and secreted proteins. And, controlled as tightly as all the actions and reactions of the organism, when its job is done, the system shuts down.

So how can it fail? Most obviously, it may fall prey to attackers *of* the immune system. Perhaps the most dramatic case in point in the 1980s is acquired immune deficiency syndrome—AIDS. Bob Gallo, among the first to isolate the virus believed to cause AIDS, would elaborate for me a whole set of characteristics that led him to believe the AIDS virus (which he dubbed HTLV-III) is a first cousin of the only known human cancer virus, human T-cell leukemia virus (HTLV-I).

But a whole range of other parasitic, viral, and bacterial diseases and cancers work by evading or crippling the immune response. Generally, these succeed because they either do not trigger the macrophages and lymphocytes, or because they somehow neutralize the antibodies or killer T-cells.

(The immune system contains other components, several recently discovered, that won't be discussed.)

Parasites have developed a fascinating array of tricks to evade immunity—tricks that may offer clues to how cancer cells do so. Some (schistosomes) actually capture and coat themselves in their host's surface markers. Others immediately move into the host's cells, where they can remain undetected by the circulating immune cells. And others, like the trypanosomes of "sleeping sickness," constantly alter their surfaces so that the antibodies elaborated against them cannot find their targets. Finally, some parasites may secrete proteins that directly destroy antibodies.

Cancer has dogged immunologists for decades. Certainly many of the surface antigens of tumor cells would not be recognized as nonself, since they are the result of one's own cells' proliferation, but there is strong evidence for the existence of some tumor-specific antigens. Perhaps, the thinking goes, their concentration is sometimes too weak to evoke a sufficiently powerful immune response. It is also possible that tumors secrete molecules that shut down the immune response. There is circumstantial evidence for every method of evasion of the immune response by tumors; it seems certain that different cancers, like different parasites, use different methods that may be more or less effective in given individuals, or at given times in a person's life.

But there is also the more dismal view. DNA is being replicated millions of times a day in every living person. Errors are bound to occur—are known to occur with a certain frequency, in fact. Therefore systemic, deadly cancer may represent simply the statistical outcropping of errors: the expected occasional case when all the immune surveillance against such errors breaks down. Dismal because this does not suggest a way out. Like the earlier beliefs that cancer may be a part of life, it suggests no cure. But it is not the prevalent view.

Michael Potter came to the National Cancer Institute in 1954, medical degree fresh in hand, and set out to help unravel the mysteries of the immune system. Then, and for several years afterward, it was not even known that lymphocytes fell into the two major classes of B and T cells, and little was known of antibodies or their method of attack. Potter has been part of so many major discoveries that tracing his career depicts the development of immunology from what he calls "the explosion" of the late 1950s to the present world of monoclonal antibodies, a kind of protein he helped create now being used experimentally in the cancer war.

In 1954 it was virtually unknown how antibodies did their job, for much the same reason that enzyme action was then little understood. There are so many antibodies, they are so specific to particular invaders, that it seemed impossible to get a handle on them, some commonality from which to proceed. Even if you could get a test tube full of antibodies, which you couldn't, they would be a mixture of thousands of different kinds. Most of Potter's early work went toward getting large copy numbers of single antibodies and purifying out quantities of single antibodies. That made it possible to elucidate the structure, a long task in which he played a major role.

This assessment is not from him but from others in the field; Potter speaks modestly of his own role. "He has always been considered a real resource in immunology," Vicki Sato says.

The mouse model, this time. Potter began working on mouse tumors, in particular a type called plasmacytomas. His partner then was Thelma Dunn, "an outstanding mouse-pathologist," he recalls, who had accurately described many mouse plasma cell tumors. This seemingly obscure work led to their discovery that certain of these tumors contained a protein in large quantity that evoked a single-antibody response; that led to the first purification of antibody protein.

Let's say the immune system needs to be capable of producing ten thousand different antibodies against that many viral and other antigens' tumor surface markers. That seems a difficult evolutionary problem, especially given that the antibodies must be tailor-made quickly to a given invading antigen. The solution turned out to be what a scientist would call "elegant": Immunoglobulin (antibody) genes all have certain constant regions, common to all, and variable regions that may contain a wide variety of different codings. The key, Potter notes, is a "retrieval system" that allows a piece of this gene to be expressed with a piece of that—a combination, in other words, that allows the creation of highly individualized proteins from relatively few templates.

"And there you have an example of the beautiful design of nature," says Potter at his desk. If you need ten thousand different immunoglobulin proteins, the simplest way to get them would be to code for a hundred of this kind and a hundred of that kind and find a retrieval system for mixing and matching, a hundred times a hundred.

For the moment, consider just these two vital revelations derived from the studies of mouse plasmacytoma: There were tumor-specific antigens, markers that allow a creature's own immune system to distinguish a tumor in the crowd of self-cells; and at least a few antibodies could be purified to study their structures.

(A chromosomal translocation was first discovered in a mouse tumor, and Potter noted that reading the report of it set Michael Cole and Grace Shen Ong on the course that led them to discover the *myc* oncogene translocated in Burkitt's lymphoma.)

Move one more step: If the body "elaborates" antibodies, literally sculpting them to fit a given invader's antigen proteins, and if tumors have *any* specific markers on the surface of their cells, then why can't we "build-to-suit" an antibody against a cancer in our laboratory?

Potter and others could get quantities of one particular antibody; the problem was, they couldn't get quantities of any antibody on demand. Each of the thousands is evoked or elaborated only for a given brief time, and then only *in vivo*. After all, the inability of normal cells to reproduce more than a few times is a key feature of the test for transformation *in vitro*. It was ultimately the British molecular biologist Cesar Millstein, building on Potter's foundation, who found the answer. The idea is simple in concept, but the creation was terrifically complex. Antibody cells are highly specific but impossible to culture in the lab. Cancer cells reproduce forever but are clonal, identical to the original. Millstein created a hybrid cell, a hybridoma, which as a cancer cell reproduced readily *in vitro*, and it produced antibody, always the same antibody. Thus at the other end of the production line he got a monoclonal antibody. Millstein and colleagues won the 1984 Nobel Prize for their landmark work. In the decade since his discovery, hybridoma or monoclonal antibody technology has become biotechnology's fastest-moving field. Of all the achievements of basic cancer research, probably none holds so much promise of being quickly transferrable into the clinic as monoclonal antibodies.

Clinical trials are already in progress around the country, targeting monoclonal antibodies developed against specific tumor antigens for a variety of purposes. First, such an antibody can be tagged with a radioactive marker so that a microtumor or micrometastasis too small to detect otherwise might be found. The antibody would home in directly on the tumor antigen and latch onto it. Second, chemotherapeutic drugs that now have devastating side effects because of their toxicity to other tissues could be linked to such antibodies and targeted directly at tumors and metastases—for metastases, remember, are clones of the original tumor, not new tumors induced in distant tissue. That would finally give chemotherapy the specificity of radiation therapy while retaining the power of chemical agents to interfere with tumor cell reproduction.

At any rate, that has been the promise since Millstein's creation of the first monoclonal antibody in 1975. The first report I heard that the promise might soon be fulfilled came on one September day, in the giant NIH hospital building, in the office of Dr. Stephen Larson.

Larson's group has already been able to detect deeper tumors than is possible with other techniques, using monoclonal antibodies developed against melanomas and colon and breast cancers. "There are frustrations," Larson says, "because there always seem to be more questions than answers." For example, although the specific antibodies have been developed, they are sometimes broken down chemically before reaching the tumors, or if they reach the tumors, they may break down before enough of them collect to be detectable.

Antibody is injected into the bloodstream, Larson says, and it gradually percolates throughout the entire body; if all goes well, it binds and collects at tumor-antigen sites. Larson noted that antibodies' protein chains have active segments attached like arms to the molecular mass. Larson's group has purified these arms alone, permitting them to inject larger amounts of active ingredient and lessening the chance of degradation. The difference is significant: They are using milligram doses, compared to other groups' micrograms—a thousandfold difference in dose.

Melanoma, though a skin cancer, metastasizes to the deep organs and brain. Larson believes the day is not far off when these metastases will be destroyed. Further, "We know what the specific antigens in colon cancer are and have good monoclonals against them. Our trials show good response in targeting colon tumors, and now we're beginning on breast cancer."

Such progress is all the more important given that breast cancer appears to be systemic from its onset, based on Bernard Fisher's results through the NSABP; that makes the ability to detect and fight metastases of paramount importance.

Frustrations aside, Larson says, "This is an exciting time to be in this field. I'm optimistic for the future, both in the diagnostic use and the treatment."

A note of optimism. But one to be followed, in a very different area of cancer research, by a cautious warning—about the virus, again. The human T-cell leukemia virus.

In 1978, Robert Gallo found the virologists' grail: a virus that caused leukemia in humans, specifically a cancer of the T-cells; the malignancy caused them to proliferate, but the infection simultaneously reduced their ability to function. The only such virus found so far, of a rare cancer, it is a fascinating little bug independent of its unique place in the cancer story.

Gallo remembers spending two years characterizing HTLV before publishing his results in 1980. He paces as he talks, the wall behind him holding bulletin boards jammed with pictures of postdoctoral fellows, colleagues, family. One wall holds awards, plaques, diplomas. And of course there is the ubiquitous white board with felt-tip pens on which he can slash straight lines (genes) or circles (plasmids) with restriction enzymes. Chief of the NCI's laboratory of tumor cell biology, he is energetic and assertive, speaks rapidly, and sometimes draws out words for emphasis much like astronomer Carl Sagan.

He finds the NCI his ideal research environment because of its catholic orientation—"Here, you go from the molecule to the man" —and he enjoys the atmosphere of large laboratories in constant interaction. He found HTLV, he says, because he refused to listen to the prevailing wisdom. But he is quick to add that in science individualism does not play the role it does in the arts.

"If Michelangelo had never lived there would be no Sistine ceiling, and if Beethoven had never lived there'd be no Ninth Symphony," he says. "But if any given scientist had never lived, I believe we'd still have found what we've found. We're like enzymes; maybe each of us makes something happen faster, and we each have our own pathway."

The argument he refused to heed is simple: In order to have transformation from a virus, you needed to have massive infection. No one had seen cancer develop without being preceded by massive viral replication. That certainly was true in mouse leukemia. Therefore, the argument went, if a virus caused a human cancer, it would have been found.

Gallo's hypothesis was that some viruses might transform cells even when present in tiny amounts, with very low expression of their transforming proteins, making them very hard to detect. The discovery of reverse transcriptase, the invention of the Southern blot, and other technological advances put tools in Gallo's hands to detect increasingly smaller amounts of virus. Finally, he found it, and soon afterward discovered a close relative, dubbing the pair HTLV-I and -II.

Now we know some viruses are "associated" with some cancers, meaning that viral infection is one step in what may be a long and complex pathway, acting as an initiator or promoter or element in either step. But did this mean that a virus had been found that *caused cancer*?

"Yes."

So this is a cancer you *catch*?

"Exactly. And people say it's rare. It's rare in the United States in 1984, but I'm not sure it's rare in other countries. This cancer has an interesting epidemiology. The virus is endemic in Jamaica and some other West Indies islands; and there's evidence that 70 percent of all adult lymphoid tumors in Jamaica involve HTLV infection."

Further, Gallo warns, he does not believe the cancer is spread from one victim to the next in the ordinary way viral infections are passed on. He believes carriers, many of whom do not get cancer, transmit it through blood transfusions and sexual relations. If that begins to sound like a relative of AIDS, acquired immune deficiency syndrome, indeed there are many similarities, to be noted soon.

Gallo has found the virus endemic in what would appear to be an eclectic group of populations: northern Africa, the Caribbean, several Pacific islands, and a few of the Japanese islands. Jewish Ethiopians have carried the virus to Israel, and it has been detected in Spain. Gallo says HTLV is very similar to a virus that infects some Old World monkeys and believes that may be the key to its epidemiology: He thinks Portuguese slave traders exported it from

Africa during a very narrow range of time, in the seventeenth century, simultaneously taking it to the Caribbean, parts of the South American coast, Macao, and finally Japan.

Some mammal viruses cause monoclonal tumors: They cause transformation very rarely, so any tumor that develops grows from a single cell. Other such viruses cause polyclonal tumors because many cells are transformed, and the resultant malignancy will represent a population of all descendants. Scientists break these viruses down into "slow" versus "fast" or "chronically transforming" versus "acutely transforming." HTLV, Gallo says, bears resemblances to both. Acutely transforming viruses contain a captured oncogene; chronically transforming viruses do not. Acutely transforming viruses transform cells *in vitro* and may not even exist in nature; chronically transforming viruses transform only *in vivo*, and certainly exist in nature. HTLV is chronically transforming but transforms *in vitro*, exists in nature yet contains an extra gene that, while not captured like an oncogene, appears tied to the virus's transforming ability.

"HTLV is a retrovirus, yet bears many similarities to DNA tumor viruses," he says. "It may be a bridge between the two."

He is disturbed that because other human cancer viruses have not been found, the *role* of viruses in cancers—Epstein–Barr in Burkitt's —has been underplayed, and he pointed out that recent evidence links another virus (papilloma) to cervical cancer.

Gallo does not believe we are facing an epidemic of HTLV-induced cancers, because the virus appears to be only moderately efficient at transformation. He does believe that the powers of its cousin, HTLV-III, the cause of AIDS, have been grossly underestimated. Perhaps out of a desire not to face the problem, he says, the homosexual connection to AIDS has been "almost voyeuristically overplayed."

Interestingly, the two viruses, so similar in molecular structure, have precisely the opposite effects on the T-cells they infect. Both I and III are fairly homologous, both are human retroviruses—retroviruses because they use reverse transcriptase to produce DNA. HTLV-I causes proliferation, but only of a tiny portion of the T-cells it infects, though it sharply reduces the ability of all infected T-cells to function in immune defense. HTLV-III kills T-cells, and it is far more efficient than -I, Gallo says. AIDS victims basically lose their immune defenses and die of opportunistic infections and such ordinarily rare cancers as Kaposi's sarcoma.

A little while later, over lunch and over a different subject, Gallo returns to a thought very much on his mind these days. "I think HTLV-III is going to be a much bigger public health problem than -I; and I'm not sure anyone is prepared to accept that."

21

Migration

Lance Liotta is a pathologist, an M.D./Ph.D. in a specialty perfect for someone with his intense basic-research interests. "I don't have to see patients every day, but I have a lot to do with patients," he says. "A pathologist remains very much part of the world of patient care, but you don't have the immediate concerns of a doctor on the ward."

Liotta's overriding concern is metastasis, and though not a "name" nationally at this point, he is a rising star here at the NCI thanks to some remarkable work he has done in tracing the strange journey of cells that have not only begun behaving like individuals rather than like cooperative members of an organism, but which have further developed the ability to move, as though purposefully, from their base anchorage point to distant parts of what has now become their host.

Liotta believes that this branch of cancer research may have real payoffs practically; that if the underlying principles of invasion and metastasis can be understood, then those deadly stages of cancer might be prevented. At that point, it would make sense to report that a microtumor had been detected somewhere in the body, even if the site were unknown, if a ready means were available to prevent the tumor's moving until it would be either destroyed by the immune system or, grown large enough, removed by irradiation or surgery.

Here is what Liotta now knows of the process. First, recall that these cellular bags of jelly are anchored to a matrix made of collagen and other strong proteins, some rigid, some elastic, depending on what the final constitution of the tissue is to be. These skeletal blocks of the intracellular matrix are responsible for much of the architecture of the tissues in which they are located. They provide anchorage for cells, and it is often through them as media that molecules are transported up to or into the cells, whether as messengers or for other purposes.

The metastatic cell must first break loose from this matrix, then degrade the collagen. In fact, Liotta has found collagenase, the enzyme that degrades that protein, in invasive tumors.

Ultimately, Liotta says, the metastatic tumor must invade the barrier of matrix that separates different tissue types; break through the wall of a blood vessel and enter the bloodstream; then survive the trauma of travel through the bloodstream or lymph system and evade or survive antibodies, killer T-cells, all the defenses of the body; now degrade the blood vessel wall to get back out; and finally lodge and thrive in some place that should be hostile to its type of cell. There its cells not only must manage to survive and reproduce, but if they grow large enough they must be able to communicate through this tissue to draw a blood supply.

Back to the beginning. The way here is step by step. "Invasive tumor cells have a deranged interaction with the matrix. Normally, the epithelium rests on a basement membrane; even benign [tumor] lesions have a basement membrane, a form of extracellular matrix that they are attached to"—a key distinction, a major change that marks to doctor or scientist the shift from a growing ball of cells to cancer. "If you damage an organ, remove some cells, they'll grow back on the basement membrane. But if the basement membrane is damaged, they can't. Not so with tumor cells."

Tumor cells break through the basement membrane. First, the tumor cells bind to the matrix, and Liotta believes he has found the key binding point, a matrix protein called laminin, shaped like a cross, for which he knows some tumors have receptors. The laminin receptor binds at the point where the molecule's arms intersect. Normal cells have all their laminin receptors filled. Tumor cells that he has studied have exposed laminin receptors that may, like magnets, draw the cells onward. Once bound to the laminin, the migrating tumor cell apparently secretes its collagenase and other degredative enzymes to degrade those cells only in its immediate vicinity—and we are now envisioning something on the microscopic level. The tumor cell then pulls itself slowly through the hole created, pseudopod fashion, the same way an amoeba and many other microbes move. It is drawn on—and Liotta is not entirely sure of the mechanism of this attraction—to the next layer of basement cells.

"This [protein-degrading] enzyme is augmented in tumor cells in which we've put the gene that makes them metastatic," he says.

You can make cells metastatic? There is a silence now, a serious pause. In the test tube?

"Certain oncogenes put in a cell colony will make it metastatic, yes. In our latest, unpublished work, we've been able to transfer DNA into recipient cells and get them to become metastatic when before they had been benign."

That work in fact would be published in the journal *Molecular and Cell Biology* in January 1985. Liotta and co-workers were able to induce metastases in nude mice by using the *n-ras* and *ras* oncogenes. There are questions: Nude mice are immune deficient. Does that, rather than the oncogenes, account for the occasional metastasis? That is, has a metastasis gene been found, or does this represent a failure in immune surveillance? Is it background, like the spontaneous transformation of cells in a focus, or is it real? But there is metastasis, and as interestingly, in these metastases Liotta has found increased expression of laminin receptors.

At the practical end of the spectrum, Liotta says some drug firms now are studying collagenase inhibitors as possible anticancer therapeutics, but this research is still very new. Agents to detect other chemicals being found associated with metastasis may also be developed, to detect cancerous invasion early enough to counterattack. And, of course, some means to counterattack must be developed— that answer may lie with monoclonal antibodies, interferon, or both. All this seems consistent with the behavior of known oncogenes, producing growth factors at inappropriate times, cells perhaps responding to the wrong growth factors because their mutated oncogenes have produced a receptor for them when none should exist.

Liotta has some doubt about the existence of a single "angiogenesis factor" as reported by Judah Folkman several years ago. Tumors can "vascularize," bring in blood vessels to nourish them. Folkman believes a single factor is responsible for this, a factor that may be activated in cancer.

But Liotta notes that vascularization, the building of new blood vessels in wounds or in tumors, "is a very complex process, and I would think the angiogenesis factor should have been purified by now, if it existed." Rather, Liotta thinks such a process is the net effect of another of the "cascades" of many genes acting in concert.

The question is, why do each of these steps occur in the perfect harmony they must for a tumor cell to move and reestablish, when harmony appears to be the most obvious missing quality in cancer? Most invading tumor cells are believed killed by the mere turbulence of the blood, for example, for virtually all but blood cells are accustomed to a relatively placid existence attached to the matrix, rather than the spinning, tumbling, high-pressure vortex within an artery.

That answer is not yet known, but Liotta believes that by studying the chemical products of metastatic tumors, working his way back to their genes, moving forward then to the next step, he may be able to isolate the gene, then the genes whose inappropriate signals spell the final message: cancer, and cancer of a particular type of tissue.

"I don't think any of these things that an invasive tumor cell does are unique. They're just throwbacks to some normal function that is used occasionally or only in the embryonic state—something that has come under very tight regulation and that has then thrown off that regulation."

The fetus: Recall that at some point in the growing ball of cells—divided only into the types ectoderm, mesoderm, endoderm—comes a signal, or a cascade of signals. Now, as in musical chairs, cells suddenly begin migrating from their natural homes to what should be their permanent ones. *Should* be. What are those migrational signals? What triggers them? Are the errors that allow the signals to be turned on again fifty years later, billions of cell divisions later, present at the creation or are they induced later on?

Still, we have metastasis in a mouse, *in vivo*, at last.

Shelly Bernstein is at work in the lab. Winter, late December 1984. Neither he nor Weinberg wants to overstate his findings, to shock anyone into false expectations. But here's what he has done—and I can't help but notice in it how every successful experiment is a reliving of so many other successful experiments. He spent months transfecting metastasized *human* tumor cells into his large colony of from 100 to 150 mice in the animal laboratory. He wanted to use mice with perfectly well-developed immune systems, rather than nude mice, but he needed to use NIH3t3 connective tissue cells in an intermediate step because they are easy to grow. Therefore, his mice are of a breed called NFS; they are genetically the closest match available to the NIH3t3 mice, and Bernstein wanted to minimize the possibility of transplant rejection by the mice's immune system, knowing there was nothing he could do to eliminate the possibility altogether because the cell line has been bred for so long.

First he broke the human DNA down into manageable fragments —not necessarily gene-sized but around 30,000 bases long, small enough to be taken up in cells. That can be done, remember, by squirting the DNA through a syringe or pipette, so enormous is the tightly bonded molecule. The shattered DNA is plated with calcium phosphate, grown up in cell cultures. Transformed cells are inoculated into the mice. (At some point, a susceptible animal has to catch this strange illness of the migratory cells, postulated Koch.)

Finally, luck. Bernstein managed to get metastatic tumors in mice that had not had them—just a couple, though, out of hundreds tried. Now he took the DNA of those tumors, broke it down, and retransfected it. Again he found metastases, but this time at a far greater rate than in the first round. That was exciting. Now the transfected DNA contained less human DNA than in the first round. As the mouse–human DNA was transfected in round after round, now recalling the early efforts in Weinberg's lab to isolate the oncogenes using the human *alu* probe, the odds would be that less human, more mouse DNA would wind up in the transfectant mix. But whenever there was metastasis, you would know that there was at least some human DNA present, and that among it was the gene or genes responsible for metastasis. In every serial transfection Bernstein located the same pieces of human DNA, their identity still unknown.

But consider: It was a small segment of human DNA. It was present in a tumor that metastasized in the human patient who was its donor. Now it had *caused* tumors to metastasize in mice. Those results were published in *Proceedings of the National Academy of Sciences* in March 1985.

Epilogue

By the fall of 1985 there were several new developments in the
oncogene story, though there are still as many answers that remain
frustratingly just beyond reach. After months of effort, Shelly Bernstein still had not been able to fully isolate and identify the gene
sequence that had caused metastasis in the benign tumors of normal
mice. Several times it seemed within grasp, only to vanish. Yet the
promise did not vanish: "We know we have a segment of DNA that
is one part of the mechanism of this metastasis," Weinberg said
recently. "But as is so often the case, what we had thought would
take three months now looks like it will take a year.

"We had thought the isolation of the gene would be straight-
forward and that we would have it sequenced by now. We thought
we had our hands on the needle in the haystack, but not quite. I
think we're on track now."

Weinberg pointed out that in the days before gene cloning, it was
enough for a scientist to demonstrate the existence of a gene. Now
in order to credibly claim to have "found" a gene, "you are under
obligation to isolate it and demonstrate the subtleties of structure,
and that's good in the long run but obviously takes more time."

The DNA Bernstein is using was isolated from a human cervical
sarcoma. Despite the delay, Weinberg said he has been encouraged
to find that "the biochemical traits of cells acquiring the gene are

251

distinctly different from those not; perhaps most significantly, these secrete large quantities of proteases"—protein-degrading enzymes, which destroy intracellular matrix tissue. Meanwhile, "cells equally tumorigenic but non-metastatic generally don't secrete proteases at all." Weinberg expected to determine the sequence of this gene by the end of 1985.

Weinberg remains more enthusiastic than ever about the implications of Land's gene-pair transformations. In Edinburgh, Demetrios Spandidos has reported transforming normal cells with *ras* alone. But to do so, all the surrounding cells that haven't taken up *ras* must be killed off; only then will the *ras*-bearing cell be transformed.

"But that says something to me about the actions of that second oncogene," *myc* in the original experiments. "The neighboring cells must be exerting an influence on the single-oncogene bearing cell that prevents its transforming. With the second, right oncogene, the cell overcomes that influence."

Discovery of the *neu* oncogene by Weinberg's lab turned out to be more exciting than expected, although major work is still to come. There Min Chie Hung and Cornelia Bargmann cloned a large gene 33,000 base-pairs in length; *neu* encodes for a heavy protein, composed of 1,500 amino acid units.

The protein's function: It is a growth factor receptor, "that much is crystal clear. It's analogous to the EGF receptor but is quite distinct from it," says Weinberg. The important unknown, however, is how the oncogene arose and what growth factor it is receptor for.

Weinberg predicts that the difference between this oncogene and its normal counterpart will turn out to be small, likely a point mutation—alteration of a single base "letter" in the gene's sequence, just as was the case between the human bladder oncogene and viral *ras*, demonstrated years earlier. "During formation of human tumors, severe rearrangements of genes are hard to find. Point mutations are much more likely in human tumors." That jibes with the action of chemical carcinogens, Weinberg says, "many of which create point mutations."

The discoveries of the past year are interesting extensions of those made earlier. Weinberg cites as "*the* discovery of 1984" the finding by Michael Wigler, announced that September, that a strain of yeast whose *ras* gene is defective is also deficient at spoor production—

reproduction. *Ras*, remember, is the gene found throughout most living things, even unicellular yeast. Wigler and a group of yeast geneticists then found that if *ras* were inserted into the defective yeast cells, they began reproducing normally. It does not appear that the normal function of *ras* in mammals is as simple as in yeast (it encodes the enzyme that synthesizes a key second messenger called cyclic AMP.) But Wigler's group appears on its way to learning what normal *ras* does in mammals; that would be a vital piece of the reductionist puzzle.

Weinberg notes that the oncogene story so far has revealed that cancer cells' growth autonomy always relates to their ability to grow "without the goading of growth factors," and such transformation is achieved in three distinct ways:

—The cancer cell secretes its own growth factors, instead of just receiving them out of the bloodstream, creating autocrine rather than endocrine growth stimulation. Now it appears that *ras* and *mos* as well as polyoma middle T all cause tumor cells to secrete transforming growth factors. *Sis*, of course, encodes platelet-derived growth factor (PDGF).

—The oncogene causes activation of a second gene that turns on transforming growth-factor genes. *Ras*, *mos*, *fes*, and *abl* as well as polyoma middle T appear able to do this. Again, the result is an autocrine loop.

—The oncogene encodes a growth-factor receptor that alters the cell constitutively. The nucleus is constantly bombarded with signals to grow even though the cell is not bathed in growth factor. Thus the cell acquires autonomy from growth factors.

Now, investigators at St. Jude's Children's Research Hospital in Memphis, Tennessee, have found that the oncogene *fms* (pronounced fems) encodes for a truncated growth-factor receptor. The normal version of this, known as CSF-1, is the growth factor receptor of macrophage cells, immune defense scavenger cells that swim through the bloodstream to engulf invading antigens and dead red blood cells. Weinberg referred to this as *"the* discovery of 1985."

Charles Sherr, chairman of tumor cell biology at St. Jude's, and Carl W. Rettenmier, assistant member of the department, made the discovery in the summer. Sherr told me that although the data show the *fms* protein is related to the CSF-1 receptor, it would take several months to determine if it in fact was a truncated version of it, as it appears to be, "truncated at both ends."

If so, Sherr said, he sees two possible modes of action. The oncogenic virus which captured *fms* causes a fibrosarcoma, a malignancy of the hormone-producing cell. Thus, the virus puts the receptor gene "into a cell that *makes* the hormone," making its action appear analogous to *sis's* yielding PDGF, "but because the receptor appears slightly truncated, it's also possible that its kinase activity might be constitutive," that is, that it might send its growth signals without outside stimulation, analogous to *erbB* and its truncated EGF.

Weinberg says all this leads him to believe that the series of steps taken by action of all oncogenes allows the cell to grow without restraint, but that the step or steps of invasion and metastasis "are fundamentally different. The ability to insinuate [into other tissue layers] and evade immune defense implies to me a different set of characteristics. Ordinarily, broken-away cells would be an easy target for immune defense. No, I think metastasis is functionally different."

Weinberg believes that each event in the further stages of cancer is an extremely rare one—an event of very low probability made likely because oncogene actions multiply the chances. If, for example, there is one chance in a million of one of these further genetic missteps leading to metastasis, then the freely growing ball of cells must only reach a clonal colony size of one million for one cell to be likely to take that misstep. "Of course, taking this step confers on that new cell a great growth advantage, and it begins multiplying rapidly to bring about the single occurrence of the next rare event in the evolution of a tumor.

"Evolution of a tumor; of course, the usual word is progression, but really, I've just been recapitulating Darwinian evolution."

Mutations occur at random. If, in the course of millions of mutations, one accidentally confers an advantage on its recipient, its descendants might even squeeze out their normal siblings. . . . And there is no advantage a single cell can acquire better than growth—reproduction—even growth at the expense of cooperation.

Back in December of 1984 Bernstein had thought that he had the metastasis gene "in hand," that it would take but a few months to corner and name the beast. But he is far from discouraged. After months of setbacks, by last summer's end he felt sure he was close, and hoped to have results by December, 1985. A long, wearying chase and not one for the impatient. Brighter news from across the river:

"Jacquelyn Manzi has been off chemotherapy treatment since spring," Bernstein said. "Her cell count and bone marrow are fine, her face is thinning. She looks and sounds terrific.

"I saw John Cabral and Patrick Gormely yesterday," August 19, 1985. "John is a year off treatment, but we had a scare Sunday. He was not feeling good; had pains in his ribs, flanks and thighs, some bruising of his legs, and that sometimes indicates that the platelets are low. But when we checked him Monday his counts were fine. I can't rule out a relapse, but I think it's just a virus. He rides a dirt bike—he's a very active kid—and that could account for the bruises."

Patrick Gormely had been worrying Bernstein because he had an outbreak of warts—present the year before, when I spoke to him. Nothing seemed to cure them. "They're virally caused, so there's always a possibility that there's an underlying disease weakening the immune system," Bernstein said. Then, days earlier, Patrick had bitten one of the warts. His mother applied an over-the-counter bandage soaked in a mild medication. The warts all disappeared.

"He's doing wonderfully," Bernstein said. "He just looks so good, a bright-smiling kid. I was so pleased."

In Tucson, surgeon Hugo Villar reported that Belinda Mims and Bob Delp both were doing well and were cancer-free some 15 months after surgery.

Perhaps the most exciting news came from Johns Hopkins University, where Dr. Stanley E. Order reported successfully treating liver cancer patients with radioactively tagged monoclonal antibodies. Advanced liver cancer has always been fatal and virtually untreatable. Order reported in August, 1985 that after treatment, tumors shrank 30 percent or more in nearly half of 104 patients in the study.

In one dramatic case, a twenty-eight-year-old woman with a tumor weighing more than five pounds—previously certainly fatal— had her tumor shrunk so far that surgeons could remove it. She appeared to be free of cancer after 15 months. Another patient whose tumor weighed 15 pounds—"the largest human cancer I have ever seen," Order told the *New York Times*—had her tumor shrunk to less than two pounds after a year's treatment.

In October, 1984, Bernstein had gotten a phone call that, while not changing his life, helped fix it in its current direction. After missing a persistent caller all day long, just as he was about to leave for the day he was reached by an executive of the MacArthur Foundation. Bernstein had been named a recipient of one of the new so-called "genius grants," a stipend that varies by individual but is said to run at least $25,000 a year for five years, tax-paid and with no restrictions on its use.

"In the case of people like me, in research, its purpose is partly to offer inducement to remain in research even though clinical practice pays a lot better," Bernstein said. He was pleased with the recognition and encouragement.

Still, he would have been where he is, chasing down narrower and narrower corridors, knowing that in this mix he forever thins there is a quantifiable amount of DNA causing tumors to migrate in laboratory mice of the NFS breed. Is this *real* metastasis he is hunting? It certainly seems so. Human metastasis or possibly a figment of the laboratory? Cancer or artifact? In a few weeks, maybe a month, maybe before you've even gotten here, Bernstein or another investigator may have isolated and purified the gene, and maybe we will know if we've found the ultimate step in the cascade to cancer. Maybe this time, bringing his mind into sharpest focus on that unseeable world, he is right on target.

Notes

Prologue

Page viii: *Its Editor, John Maddox . . . second to none in the world.* John Maddox, interview, and opening remarks, Molecular Biology of Cancer conference, Boston, Mass., Sept. 10, 1984.

Page ix: *Some two hundred forms . . . have been distinguished. Cancer: Science and Society,* Cairns, John C., P. 22.

Page x: *Down through the ages . . . evolution of an idea.* "The Contribution of Recent NSABP Clinical Trials of Primary Breast Cancer Therapy to an Understanding of Tumor Biology—An Overview of Findings," Fisher, Bernard, M.D., et al., CANCER, Vol. 46, No. 4, August 15, 1980.

Chapter 1

Page 3: *Mid-January . . . it will work.* Robert A. Weinberg interviews, July 9, 1984 and August 29, 1984, Cambridge, Mass.

Page 8: *As Weinberg put it, . . . genes of higher animals.* Weinberg interview, July 3, 1984.

Page 8: *They believed . . . mammalian cells.* Michael Wigler interview, Aug. 9, 1984, Cold Spring Harbor, N.Y.

Page 9: *necessary . . . to run your laboratory.* Weinberg interview, July 9, 1984.

Page 11: *George Khoury . . . new trend.* George Khoury interview, Sept. 6, 1984, Bethesda, Md.

Pages 11–12: *It was in chemical . . . from one mammalian cell to another.*

Weinberg interview July 9, 1984. For Weinberg's own more technical account of the oncogene story see "A Molecular Basis of Cancer, *Scientific American*, November, 1983."

Page 14: . . . *and Michael Wigler recalled that he and others turned sharply away from that avenue . . . tainted by scandal.* Wigler interview, Aug. 9, 1984.

Page 17: *Not off the wall . . . no application whatever to human cancer.* Weinberg interview, July 30, 1984, Cambridge, Mass.

Page 20: *So you put . . . laboratory dish?* Wigler interview previously cited.

Chapter 2

Page 29: *I wanted to see something.* David Baltimore, telephone interview, December, 1981.

Page 30: *I keep thinking . . . I'm going to make it.* Belinda Mims, interview, May 21, 1984, Tucson, Ariz.

Pages 32–33: *Down the hall . . . price to pay.* Robert and Vaughn Delp interview, May 21, 1984, Tucson, Ariz.

Page 33: *Villar first suspected . . . other doctors in the network.* Hugo Villar interview, May 21, 1984, Tucson, Ariz.

Pages 33–34: *As in Delp's case . . . on the tumor.* Robert Delp interview, May 21, 1984.

Pages 34–35: *Dr. Stephen Jones . . . very much related to that idea.* Stephen Jones interview, July 5, 1983, Tucson, Ariz.

Page 36: *What is bothering Villar . . . very low.* Hugo Villar interview, May 15, 1984.

Pages 36–37: *For example, the noted cancer biologist and writer John Cairns . . . would be figured into the percentages.* Cairns, John, *op. cit.* p. 151 and John Cairns interview, Aug. 27, 1984, Boston, Mass.

Page 37: *Cairns further notes . . . the United States in the past 35 years.* Cairns, *op. cit.* p. 153.

Page 37: *But you know . . . , he says bluntly.* Hugo Villar interview, May 21, 1984.

Page 37: *one critical medical oncologist . . . poor lady die.* Craig I. Henderson interview, August 30, 1984, Boston, Mass.

Chapter 3

Page 43: *Dr. Lewis Thomas . . . harm to result.* Thomas, Lewis C., *Lives of a Cell*, p. 86.

Page 46: *Gary Gallick . . . be specific.* Gary Gallick and class interview, May 31, 1984, Houston, Texas.

Page 50: *Gutterman . . . critically ill patients.* Jordan Gutterman interview, June 1, 1984, Houston, Texas.

Page 51: *The first person . . . without explanation. Ibid.*

Page 52: *The physical plant . . . 507 beds. Briefing Book*, The University of Texas System Cancer Center, Fifth Revision, February, 1984, pp. 20–23; Sixth Revision, May, 1985, pp. 17–20.

Page 52: *It is only one of twenty . . . clinical cancer centers.* National Cancer Institute fact sheet.

Page 53: *Dr. Freireich . . . medical oncology.* Emil J. Freireich interview, June 1, 1984, Houston, Texas.

Page 58: *Weinberg . . . problems I study.* Robert Weinberg interview, August 29, 1984.

Page 58: *Later, Freireich . . . hence the dilemma, sui generis.* Emil J. Freireich telephone interview, June 20, 1985.

Chapter 4

Page 60: *Michael Wigler . . . interesting problem.* Michael Wigler interview, August 9, 1984.

Pages 63–64: *Unfortunately . . . taken too seriously.* Robert Weinberg interview, July 9, 1984.

Chapter 5

Page 67: *George Khoury . . . Massachusetts General Hospital.* George Khoury interview, Sept. 6, 1984, Bethesda, Md.

Page 73: *Weinberg noted . . . cancerous transformation.* Robert Weinberg interview, July 30, 1984.

Page 76: Weinberg recalls of the "horse race" on discovering the point mutation that his and Barbacid's labs made the discovery at virtually the same moment.

Page 77: *Weinberg says . . . influenced the graduate student. Ibid.*

Chapter 6

Page 84: *For Hartmuth Land . . . March 1982.* Hartmuth Land interview, June 26, 1984, Cambridge, Mass.

Pages 84–85: *Parada . . . good fortune.* Luis Parada interview, June 26, 1984, Cambridge, Mass.

Page 85: *Arriving in . . . skeptical of. Ibid.*

Page 87: *Weinberg recalls . . . in his mind.* Robert Weinberg telephone interview, March 13, 1985.

Page 88: *Parada recalls . . . through its paces.* Luis Parada interview, August 15, 1984.

Page 92: *Land calls this . . . pass it along.* Hartmuth Land interview, July 15, 1984.

Page 93: *In choosing . . . in the long run.* Robert Weinberg interview, August 29, 1984.

Page 95: *We measure the tumor . . . die quickly, he says.* Luis Parada interview, June 26, 1984.

Page 96: *Swashbucklers . . . Sidney Farber.* Emil Frei interview, July 12, 1984, Boston, Mass.

Chapter 8

Page 101: *Weinberg . . . And the rest is history.* Robert Weinberg interview, July 29, 1984. The scientists cited are Minoo Rassoulzadegan and Francois Cuzin of Nice, France, and A. Van der Eb of the Netherlands.

Chapter 9

Pages 109–110: Song "Vanishing Species," written by Joanne Cipolla, copyright 1983, Fishweasel Music.

Chapter 10

Page 111: *Monday . . . ten hours.* Hartmuth Land interview, June 26, 1984.

Chapter 11

Pages 119–120: Shelly Bernstein, interview August 16, 1984, Boston, Mass.

Page 121: *half of all childhood cancers . . . ALL. CANCER: A Manual for Practioners,* American Cancer Society Massachusetts Division, Sixth Edition, 1982. pp. 36, 297.

Page 121: *Frei himself . . . at such talk.* Emil Frei interview, July 12, 1984.

Page 122: *The speed and certainty . . . neutrally beige.* Craig Henderson interview, August 30, 1984.

Page 123: *Despite this general knowledge . . . active mind.* Emil Frei interview, July 12, 1984.

Page 124: *That leads in turn . . . have to accept it.* George Canellos interview, August 28, 1984, Boston, Mass.

Page 124: *And Craig Henderson . . . but they are important.* Craig Henderson interview, August 30, 1984.

Pages 124–125: *The second youngest . . . inquires about him.* Shelly Bernstein, Anne Manzi, Jacquelyn Manzi interview, August 20, 1984, Boston, Mass.

Page 127: *John Cabral . . . quick precision.* Shelly Bernstein, John Cabral, Aldina Cabral interview, August 20, 1984, Boston, Mass.

Page 128: *Steve Woodcheke . . . three daughters.* Steve Woodcheke, Nancy Woodcheke interview, August 20, 1984, Boston, Mass.

Page 130: *Patrick Gormely . . . acute head-inquiry clinic.* Shelly Bernstein, Patrick Gormely, Sandra Gormely, Richard Gormely interview, August 27, 1984, Boston, Mass.

Chapter 12

Page 137: *James Watson . . . occur in the cell.* Recombinant DNA: A Short Course, Watson, James D.; Tooze, John; Kurtz, David T., Scientific American Books, distributed by W. H. Freeman and Co., New York, 1983.

Page 145: *At Dana-Farber . . . explosively fast.* George Canellos interview, July 12, 1984.

Page 146: *The Wihtehead Institute . . . 14 years old.* Nature, August, 1984.

Chapter 13

Page 147: *Weinberg . . . over the past six months.* Robert Weinberg interview, August 29, 1984.

Page 148: *However, of some $2 billion . . . 10 percent.* National Cancer Program: 1986 Budget Estimate to OMB pamphlet, September 15, 1984.

Page 150: *Weinberg says of the accounting . . . certain one.* Robert Weinberg interview, August 29, 1984.

Pages 150–151: *His experience . . . play it safe.* Michael Kriegler interview, July 7, 1984, Fox-Chase, Pennsylvania.

Page 155: *At the NCI . . . were being funded.* National Cancer Institute Public Information Office, telephone interview, August 22, 1985.

Page 155: *The Cancer Letter,* Jerry Boyd, Reston, Virginia, telephone interview, September 26, 1984.

Page 156: *Consider these funding figures . . . National Institutes of Health.* And further references to NCI funding all from National Cancer Program: 1986 Budget Estimate to OMB, op. cit.

Pages 157–158: *In other words . . . to cover $70,000.* Lewis Cantley, interviews with various sources.

Chapter 15

Page 166: "Oncogenes Come of Age," J. Michael Bishop, *Cell,* p. 1018, Vol. 32, April, 1983.

Page 169: Waterfield remarked on the homology at the same time in the same issue of Nature.

Page 170: *We're just writing it up . . . immortalize cells.* Hartmuth-Land telephone interview, March 13, 1985.

Pages 170, 172: *Michael Wigler . . . step two transforms.* Michael Wigler interview, August 9, 1984.

Page 172: *However, Weinberg . . . ras and a myc.* Robert Weinberg telephone interview, March 13, 1985.

Page 174: *Already I had been able . . . wrong conclusions.* Shelly Bernstein telephone interview, May 3, 1985.

Pages 175–176: *That is on Land's mind . . . but in the end it pays off.* Hartmuth Land interview, August 31, 1984, Cambridge, Mass.

Pages 176–177: *Parada agrees . . . cancer research.* Luis Parada interview, August 31, 1984, Cambridge, Mass.

Chapter 16

Page 179: *Roberts has worked . . . big T and little t.* Tom Roberts telephone interview, October 3, 1984.

Chapter 17

Pages 194–195: *Blake Cady, surgeon, is ruminating . . . secrets of cancer.* Blake Cady interview, August 27, 1984, Brookline, Massachusetts.

Page 198: *Why can we cure Hodgkin's . . . do at that point?* George Canellos interview, August 28, 1984.

Page 199: *Craig Henderson . . . watch her die.* Craig Henderson interview, August 31, 1984.

Page 206: *John Cairns . . . those numbers.* John Cairns interview, August 27, 1984, Boston, Mass.

Page 208: *Cancer rates . . . cancer as any American. Cancer: Science and Society, op. cit.* See also: *Decade of Discovery: Advances in Cancer Research 1971–1981*, NIH Publication No. 81-2323, October 1981.

Chapter 18

Page 210: *1975, and Mike Kriegler . . . he right colleagues.* Michael Kriegler interviews, July 7 and September 8, 1984, Fox Chase, Pennsylvania.

Chapter 19

Page 217: *The lady . . . treatment to follow.* Craig Henderson interview, August 31, 1984.

Page 220: *Cancer Letter Editor Jerry Boyd . . . results of it.* Jerry Boyd telephone interview, September 26, 1984.

Page 221: *To understand . . . had to participate.* "Winds of Change in Clinical Trials—from Daniel to Charlie Brown," Fisher, Bernard, M.D., reprinted in *Controlled Clinical Trials*, 4: 65–73, 1983.

Page 223: *It was Fisher who pointed out that Cancer . . . eighteenth century.* "The Contribution of Recent NSABP Clinical Trials of Primary Breast Cancer Therapy to an Understanding of Tumor Biology— An Overview of Findings," Fisher, Bernard, M.D., et al., CANCER, Vol. 46, No. 4, August 15, 1980.

Pages 223–225: References to Fisher's views on Halsted Radical Mastectomy all from previously cited CANCER article.

Page 224: *Henderson and Canellos . . . near the outset.* "Cancer of the Breast: The Past Decade," Henderson, Craig I., M.D. and Canellos, George P., M.D. *New England Journal of Medicine*, 302:17–30, January 3 and January 10, 1980.

Page 226: *The companion articles by Fisher . . . reported.* "Five-Year Results of a Randomized Clinical Trial Comparing Total Mastectomy and Segmental Mastectomy With or Without Radiation in the Treatment of Breast Cancer," and "Ten-Year Results of a Randomized Clinical Trial Comparing Radical Mastectomy and Total Mastectomy With or Without Radiation," Fisher, Bernard, M.D., et al., *New England Journal of Medicine*, 312:11, March 14, 1985.

Page 228: *In a talk . . . from the clinic.* "Laboratory and Clinical Research in Breast Cancer—A Personal Adventure," The David A. Karnofsky Memorial Lecture, Fisher, Bernard, M.D., Reprinted in CANCER RESEARCH, 40:3863–3874, November, 1980.

Page 228: *Nevertheless, Fisher later told me . . . supermarket throwaways.* Bernard Fisher telephone interview, August 23, 1985.

Chapter 20

Pages 229–230: Rachel Henderson telephone interview, May 28, 1985.

Page 237: *Michael Potter . . . cancer war.* Michael Potter interview, September 7, 1984, Bethesda, Maryland.

Page 240: *The first report . . . Dr. Stephen Larson.* Stephen Larson interview, September 6, 1984, Bethesda, Maryland.

Page 241: *In 1978 . . . cancer story.* Robert Gallo interview, September 7, 1984, Bethesda, Maryland.

Chapter 21

Page 245: *Lance Liotta . . . on the ward.* Lance Liotta interviews June 6 and September 6, 1984.

Page 249: *Shelly Bernstein . . . bred for so long.* Shelly Bernstein, telephone interview, December 27, 1984.

Epilogue

Page 251: *We know we have a segment of DNA . . . will take a year.* Robert Weinberg telephone interview, August 23, 1985.

Page 253: *Now, investigators at St. Jude's Children's Research Hospital . . . dead red blood cells.* Charles Sherr telephone interview, August 23, 1985.

Pages 254–255: *Bernstein thought . . . across the river.* Shelly Bernstein, telephone interviews, August 19 and August 22, 1985.

Page 255: *New York Times*, August 14, 1985, p. 10.

Index